"Although this book is of greatest value for those who are directly affected by childhood cancer, the well-informed and insightful account Ms. Fromer provides will instruct anyone who is at all interested in cancer."

Sanford Leiken, M.D., former chief of Pediatric Hematology-Oncology, Children's National Medical Center, Washington, DC

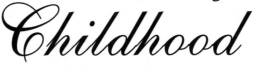

Surviving Childhood Cancer

A Guide for Families

Margot Joan Fromer

New Harbinger Publications

Distributed in the U.S.A. by Publishers Group West; in Canada by Raincoast Books; in Great Britain by Airlift Book Company, Ltd.; in South Africa by Real Books, Ltd.; in Australia by Boobook; and in New Zealand by Tandem Press.

Copyright © 1995, 1998 by Margot Joan Fromer
New Harbinger Publications, Inc.
5674 Shattuck Avenue
Oakland, CA 94609

First hardcover edition published 1995 by the American Psychiatric Press.
First paperback edition 1998.

Cover design and illustration by Lightbourne Images, copyright 1997.

Library of Congress Catalog Card Number: 97-75471
ISBN 1-57224-102-0

New Harbinger Publications' Web site address: www.newharbinger.com.

First Printing

This book is for
BRANDY SOLOMON,
for whom mere thanks
are not enough.

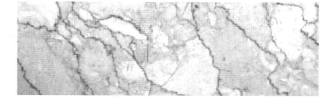

Contents

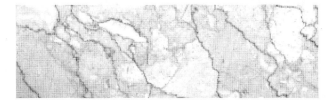

Acknowledgments

Grateful acknowledgment is made to the following: Dr. Sanford Leikin, who provided the idea and the original impetus for the book; Brandy Solomon, L.C.S.W.; Lucy Gritzmacher; and the Candlelighters Childhood Cancer Foundation.

Special and most profound thanks go to the survivors and their families who agreed to share their experiences with me. Their courage, and the positive way they faced the challenge of childhood cancer, were a source of joy and inspiration to me—as I hope they will be to the readers of this book.

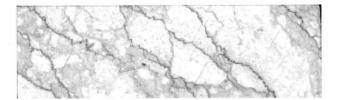

Preface

Childhood cancer is no longer an automatic death sentence. Many children now survive who once would have died. In fact, almost 70% of the children who get cancer are cured.

Cancer is the second leading cause of death among Americans under age 15. About 8,000 new cases are diagnosed each year, and one in every nine Americans under the age of 35 will be a survivor of childhood cancer. As survival improves, the death rate is less reflective of the incidence rate—that is, more children get cancer than die of it. Since 1950, the death rate has been halved.

It is tempting to turn away from thoughts of childhood cancer because it is so sad. What worse blow can fate deal to a family than the suffering of a child?

However, much of the suffering blossoms into renewed health, and most children say that not only can the pain and discomfort be borne, but there are worse things than having had cancer. Almost all of them come out of the experience stronger and better people.

It is tempting to believe that these children, especially the very little ones, do not have the strength or the will to fight off the disease. But they do. Children, perhaps even more than adults, have the stamina and determination to see the treatment through to its successful conclusion. Those who survive do so with grace and strength, and then look back on the experience and marvel at what they were able to do. They then use that newfound strength to tackle life's other challenges. They see having had cancer as a positive turning point. They don't want to be pitied, and they don't want to dwell on the illness that has passed, even though the fact of having had cancer remains with them always.

It is tempting to believe that, although a child has won the battle against cancer, the emotional and physical costs of the treatment were so high that in the end the struggle wasn't worth it. It would seem logical to question the value of survival under these terms, but this is not so. It is true that some children are left with physical or mental limitations, but they adjust to them and are able to go on to future happiness and productive lives.

It is tempting to believe the myth that families crack and break apart under the stress of childhood cancer. Some parents who before the illness struck were already on the verge of divorce do not manage to stay together, but most do. In fact, families usually draw closer together as a result of this brush with death and the suffering of one of their members. People have more strength and emotional durability than they—or others—give them credit for.

It is tempting to believe that children who have had cancer can never draw another anxiety-free breath, that they are perpetually worried about recurrence, even years later, and that they walk through life under the sword of Damocles. This is not true. Sometimes the cancer does reappear, and even though they know that they are at a somewhat higher risk for another type of cancer, the children do not grow up to become chronic worriers.

This is not to say that these young survivors do not face reality, but fear of the future is not a constant. They don't take the cancer into account every time they make a decision. Most want to be done with doctors, hospitals, and treatments. They want to leave sickness behind and get on with their lives, and they have been successful at this.

Many have a special view of the world—by and large, a healthier, more positive, and more sensitive one than the rest of us—because they *know* what's important and what's not. They know they're not invincible, and that knowledge tends to free them from shallowness and superficiality. Children who have had cancer are more independent than those who have never had to face that challenge, and they are more aware of what they want from life.

Their parents and siblings change, too, usually for the better. There is something about having faced and escaped from the ultimate grief that crystallizes values.

Children who survive cancer say that they maintained a strong sense of hope all through the treatment. This does not mean that they were not sad, even depressed, sometimes. It does, however, mean that they always thought they would get better. Hope makes it possible to consent to and continue with sometimes painful and toxic treatments. It refuses to let one give up and it prevents one from wallowing in self-pity for more than a little while at a time.

Even though childhood cancer is not in itself a positive experience, surviving it is. These young people do not live with the concept of a limited existence, and almost all say they would go through treatment again if they had to.

If one of the definitions of survival is to have experienced something dreadful, to have coped with it in a positive way, and to then be able to go on to present and future happiness, then these young people are successful survivors.

There is no recipe for survival, but there *are* ways to make the experience of cancer more bearable. These ways will be described through the stories of those who have survived the ordeal.

This book is intended for children who have the disease and for their families. Not just mothers and fathers, but brothers and sisters too, for they are as severely affected—in a different way—as the patients themselves. It is also for grandparents, aunts, uncles, and friends.

And since this is a book filled with practical help, it draws on the resources of the people who help: doctors, nurses, social workers, therapists, psychologists, and all the others who work for the survival of children with cancer.

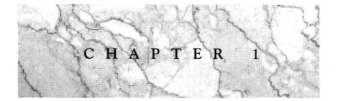

CHAPTER 1

The Diagnosis

Shock

Children are the most cherished and vulnerable members of a family, and when one of them becomes ill with a life-threatening disease, the entire family is thrown into a state of shock.

All parents have hopes, dreams, and expectations for their children. Some want them to be neurosurgeons, some have fantasies of their children having a political future, others dream that their children will be the first in the family to graduate from college. Fathers often dream of sports heroes; mothers may envision a future opera star or prima ballerina. Some dreams are less grandiose—a good job, a loving spouse, and a house full of grandchildren.

But when cancer strikes, those expectations are shattered the moment the physician utters the dread word. The reality of a kid in torn jeans swinging from his knees on a tree limb in the backyard (and his mother worrying that he'll fall and break his arm) quickly dissolves into a pale, frightened little boy alone in a hospital bed with tubes sticking into him all over.

The future Babe Ruth suddenly has only one leg; the would-be doting grandmother finds out that her daughter or son may be permanently sterile as a result of treatment. The parents of the junior-class president suddenly have a vision of the future U.S. Senator in a white coffin with weeping high school classmates grouped around the open grave.

Shock can lead to disorientation and confusion—and to an almost paralyzing difficulty in making decisions. At first, the emotional reaction to hearing a diagnosis of cancer is entirely negative. Anne Dente, a social worker at Children's Hospital National Medical Center in Washington, D.C., describes how most parents react to the news: "It's as if they had suffered a physical blow. One mother said she felt like she had been hit with a baseball bat. Another said it felt like being run over by a truck. One man said he went into the doctor's office with the suspicion that something was very wrong with his child and thought he was prepared, but when he actually heard the diagnosis, he had the sensation of being slapped."

This numbness and sense of physical assault wears off—because nature doesn't allow shock to last indefinitely and because people have to begin to cope, to accept the diagnosis, and to mobilize emotional forces.

Parents eventually learn to get on with their lives. When asked how they manage to do this, how they get out of bed in the morning, cook breakfast, take care of their other children, and just keep going while they are in the first throes of grief, Kathy Connell, another social worker at Children's Hospital in Washington, said, "I don't think they ever lead their regular lives again. They never again enjoy the same kind of normalcy that they had before their child got sick."

The lives of parents whose children have cancer are not necessarily impaired, but they *are* changed—forever. Even after the child is cured. "I don't think it's ever the same, because most of them have never experienced anything like being told that their life or their child's life might be taken. That kind of threat changes priorities," said Connell.

What gets them through it?

"Lots of things," she replied. "Their psychological makeup; how they've handled crisis in the past; religion for some people; emotional support—the relationship with their spouse, extended family, and friends; being bright and able to intellectualize the experience; and how they're treated at the hospital."

Connell also said that most parents experience an improved sense of the fullness of life and the importance of family. They come to understand the real meaning of money and possessions. "They reorder their priorities."

Parents eventually get over the shock and learn to control other emotions. They begin to make treatment decisions, and they are able to care for their sick child.

When asked how they manage to do that, what the *exact* psychological process is, Dente said, "I don't fully understand the inner workings of it, but I think parents amaze themselves at how they are able to rally. Even the families who have the most minimal resources in terms of brains or money or education seem to find the strength. I think the whole system of making decisions and getting started quickly pushes them into action so they *have* to function. The primary motivation for pulling themselves together is the child. They may want to collapse and wallow in their sorrow, but they can't do that, so they keep going."

Connell thinks that one of the reasons parents are able to deal with the illness is that the cancer is not happening to *them*. Although it is happening to a child *of* their own bodies, it is *not* their bodies that the cancer is attacking. Thus, they cannot ignore it; they have to face what's happening and carry on so the child will survive. Many of the parents interviewed for this book echoed that thought.

She added, "All the families say that they never anticipated that they could face what they are now facing and never thought they could make the decisions they are now making. But they do it because they're committed to the child's survival."

Dr. William Licamele, a child and adolescent psychiatrist at Georgetown University Medical Center in Washington, D.C., says that the best predictor of how families will react to and cope with the shock of childhood cancer is the way in which they have dealt with previous crises. "If the family is essentially chaotic and has poor coping skills, they will not do as well with cancer as families that have been able to come through intact from other bad situations."

Stress

Upon receipt of news as horrifying as childhood cancer, reality is shattered. Nothing is the way it was before—nor will it ever be again. The stress falls suddenly like a heavy blanket that seems ready to smother those who lie beneath it.

Almost without exception, this is the worst stress that a family has ever faced—and probably will ever face. It is a family illness; no one is unaffected. It is unsettling because the outcome is unknown, and it is disruptive because the normal patterns of life will not be the same for years.

All of this causes stress of the most severe sort.

A number of factors affect parents' level of stress. The child's age at diagnosis is one of the most important. Children younger than 4 and older than 7 seem to engender the most parental stress. This is because, first, little children under the age of 4 are seen as terribly vulnerable and still in need of constant protection even when they are well. In addition, they do not understand what is happening to them, which makes parents feel even more helpless as they watch their babies suffer without being able to do anything for the pain, or explain what is happening, or tell them when it will be over. Second, children who are older than 7 have moved out of the home to some extent and are developing rapidly increasing independence. They go to school alone, they have their own circle of friends, and they have a social and academic life. Therefore, serious illness is highly disruptive and drastically alters these children's lives.

Family background and socioeconomic status seem to have little bearing on reactions to the stress of childhood cancer. Nor do parents' ages, religion, or amount of education.

Familiarity with medicine and with the way the health care system functions does, however, affect the amount of stress. Suddenly, parents are thrust into a world of incredibly high technology where the principal players speak what amounts to a foreign language—and often don't bother to translate for the uninitiated. Hospitals are complex social systems that seem bent on maintaining as much secrecy as possible and separating the professional personnel from the "outsiders": patients and their families. These experiences are disconcerting, frightening, often maddening—and always stressful.

People's confidence in their ability to navigate the complexities of modern life diminishes upon setting foot in a hospital. When that confidence is further undermined by fear, shock, and every other powerful emotion that accompanies the diagnosis of childhood cancer, the result can be almost paralyzing stress.

Families need immediate help to minimize the stress—someone to help them sort through priorities: which decisions have to be made right now and which can be postponed for a while. Most parents require assistance in juggling the tasks of maintaining a household (which may include other children) and a job or two, while at the same time spending time in the hospital with the sick child. If the family lives miles from the treatment center, the logistical problems of travel, and its attendant costs, add to the stress.

It is difficult, painful, and stressful to bare one's most private thoughts and fears, especially in the midst of a crisis. But this is what happens when parents discuss treatment options with physicians who, the day before the diagnosis, were total strangers. Instant intimacy and trust make most people uncomfortable, but establishing such a relationship with health care providers is essential to the child's health and life.

Most of us prefer to cry in private, or in the company of only those who are closest to us. So when tears gush forth in public and unexpected places, the embarrassment adds to the stress of the pain and fear.

One father told this story: "I went to the hospital alone one evening a few days after Sally was diagnosed. I sat with her for a long time. She'd had chemo that morning and had spent hours retching and sweating and feeling awful. She felt better in the evening, so I read to her from *Babar the Elephant* and finally she fell asleep.

"I didn't feel like going home right away. I don't know—I just wasn't ready for my wife and Jill, my other daughter. I wasn't mad at them or anything. I guess I needed to be alone for a while, or at least away from them.

"Anyway, I was hungry, so I went to the hospital cafeteria and got something to eat—I don't even remember now what it was—and took the tray over to an empty table. I had a swallow of coffee, and then, before I had any idea what was happening, I burst into these wild tears. It was awful, sitting there in that dismal place crying my eyes out.

"Part of me was humiliated, breaking down in front of a roomful of strangers like that, but another part of me just didn't care anymore. I covered my face with my hands—I think people do that naturally when they cry—and when the storm finally subsided, I sort of peeked out from between my fingers, and there was this man sitting at my table. He was 50ish and nicely dressed in a sports jacket. There was nothing really special about him, just that he looked like a nice guy. He never said anything, but when I was finally done crying, he patted me on the shoulder. His touch was more like a woman's than like a locker-room sort of 'guy' thing.

"That was it. He gave me that pat and got up and left the table. I sat there for a while and actually ate some of that hospital food—whatever it was. I was really hungry.

"And you know what the strangest part of the whole thing was? That night, my wife and I made love for the first time since Sally got sick and it was really beautiful. Like when we were young, only better because we're not that young anymore."

This man never told his wife what happened that evening in the hospital cafeteria, and perhaps he never will. He had long since "forgiven" himself for crying in public, but keeping the experience private apparently reduced the stress he felt at the time and has added to its meaning over the years.

Emotional stress can exact a high price from parents, siblings, and other family members. All interpersonal relationships are strained. Marriages are put to a test that neither partner has had to face before.

Stress that arises from interpersonal relationships generally falls into two categories: the first as a result of what someone has said or done (for instance, making demands that are perceived as unreasonable or too difficult, blaming a spouse for the child's illness, betraying a confidence in the course of obtaining medical or psychological help), and the second as a result of what someone has *not* done (for example, refusing requested help, withholding love and attention, being unable to perform expected tasks).

Yet none of these "ancillary" stressors has the magnitude of impact that the plain fact of the cancer itself imposes. The reason is simple but far from obvious: When the life of a loved one is threatened, nothing else matters as much. One's spouse, other children, parents—all fade into relative degrees of temporary insignificance while the sick child's life is at stake.

When the immediate medical crisis has passed and the child is responding well to treatment, many of the stressful feelings that were put "on hold" come flooding back and can create problems far greater than they would have if they had not been put off.

Another man said that about a month after his son's diagnosis and leg amputation for osteogenic sarcoma, he pulled into his driveway and noticed that the grass was "practically up to my ankles." It had not occurred to him to even think about doing yard work. Mowing the lawn had been his son's chore.

"I just flipped out," he said. His next-door neighbor's perfectly manicured yard enraged him. "I went to the guy's door and instead of ringing the bell, I pounded so hard that I felt the door shake on its hinges. Then I reamed him out for being an insensitive slob and not caring about me or my family. I really felt as if he could have cut the grass—or at least have come over and offered to do it.

"I used some incredibly bad language and the guy was understandably ticked off at my effrontery. I apologized later, and he said he understood, but things have never been the same between us."

Initial Tasks

Telling a child that he or she has cancer is one of the hardest things that parents will ever have to do. They dread it, but they cannot postpone the task because once the diagnosis has been made, treatment must begin immediately.

Children respond in a variety of ways. Some demonstrate optimism and strength that is not at all manufactured. Some feel that they have to be brave so as not to upset their parents. Others exhibit passive resignation and are convinced that they are on the brink of death. Some deny the facts and go to great lengths to explain away their physical symptoms.

Any or all of these reactions can be useful coping strategies as long as they are not carried to extremes. For example, hope and strength are essential if a child (or anyone, for that matter) is to recover from a life-threatening illness. But to be constantly cheerful and to force smiles in the midst of wrenching sickness is to lose contact with reality. The child must be given the opportunity to be sad, to grieve for the way he or she was and never will be again, to rage against what has happened, and to sob out the anger and fear. The need to do this—to begin the emotional healing process—is as important, in its own way, as treating the physical disease.

Breaking the News

Many parents dread telling their child about the cancer so much that they never do it, instead allowing the child to find out "by mistake." Others believe that it is kinder to withhold reality so that their child will not become depressed. This is not a good idea.

Research has shown that the best approach to the subject of cancer is truth. The child already knows—or will soon find out—that something is seriously wrong, and a lie from the parents will then seem a betrayal. Children sense when something is drastically amiss, and even if they don't talk about it or ask questions, they imagine all sorts of horrifying things, almost all of them worse than the reality.

Yes, children will be upset and frightened. Cancer is an upsetting and frightening thing. They have every right to be scared out of their wits—for a while. The most important thing for parents is to help the child get these feelings out in the open and deal with them. It is not helpful to ignore the child's fear or to imply that it is bad or babyish or wrong in any way.

Chesler and Barbarin (1987) have described two different approaches to telling a child about a cancer diagnosis: the protective approach and the open approach. The protective approach shields both the child and his or her siblings from the full extent of reality. Advocates of this approach say that too much detailed information about the disease increases anxiety and fear, which does not lead to effective coping. Moreover, they state, families should strive for an atmosphere of normalcy, which would be disrupted by the "intrusiveness" of the illness.

Health professionals who work with children with cancer and their families are much more likely to advocate the open approach. They say that protection from truth does not calm anxiety and may in fact increase the fear that is communicated directly from parents. False cheerfulness is one of the most transparent of emotions, and lack of candor about what is really going on does not enhance honest communication within a family.

Even if one could make a good case for withholding all or part of the information from a child, attempting to do so is usually unsuccessful. Other children in the hospital will soon burst the bubble of ignorance, or the child him- or herself will make an effort to root out the truth. Siblings also play a role here. They report directly to the sick child what they have heard from schoolmates or from friends' parents—and much of what they hear (and understand) is distorted or just plain wrong. Children of elementary-school age and older can be amazingly inventive when it comes to ferreting information from a wide variety of sources: they look at their own charts, they listen to adults' conversations, they read labels on medicine containers, they look up things in the library, they quiz one another, they draw inferences from their physicians' specialties and from the procedures that are performed on them and their fellow patients.

In short, they find out what they want and need to know—and then, if their parents are not open with them, they are faced with the problem of what to do with that information. Children who have cancer are sufficiently burdened without having to take on the added responsibility of "protecting" their own parents by not talking about what is bothering them most.

Once in a while, if the parents refuse to or cannot do it, a doctor and/or social worker will join with the parents to break the news, discuss the diagnosis and treatment, and answer the child's questions. The best approach, however, is for the parents to be alone with the child in a private place and with an unlimited amount of time.

On rare occasions, parents will not be able to control the nature and amount of information that a child receives, usually when he or she is hospitalized.

Something like this happened to Rose. She had had surgery to remove a synovial cell sarcoma from her abdomen while she was in boarding school in North Carolina. Until the time the tumor was sent to the pathology lab, no one suspected cancer. Neither she nor her parents had been prepared for anything more serious than an operation to remove an odd growth. She was 16 at the time, a junior in high school.

When the pathology report revealed the cancer, Rose was sent immediately to Memorial Sloan-Kettering in New York, where she had more surgery, this time to remove surrounding tissue and lymph nodes. "My father had to go back to North Carolina to work," she said. "But I had an aunt in New York, so my mother was able to be with me the whole time I was in the hospital. For the first 3 days she stayed all day and all night, and then when I started feeling better and could get out of bed, she slept at my aunt's and wasn't at my bedside all the time.

"One day, when I was starting to think about going home, this strange doctor came into my room. My mother wasn't there, and I had never seen him before. He told me what his name was, but he said it fast and I didn't catch it. Then he told me that I would need chemotherapy."

Rose had no idea what chemotherapy meant—it's not part of an ordinary 16-year-old girl's vocabulary. "He talked real fast and told me all the bad things about chemo—the nausea, the throwing up, the things it might do to my blood, how tired I would be, how sick I would feel, and that all my hair would fall out.

"Then at the end, he stood up and told me he was moving to California—and he walked out of my room."

This physician never told Rose that the chemotherapy was designed to cure the cancer, he never smiled, he never said that the side effects were almost all temporary. He mentioned none of the things that could be done to soften the nasty effects of the drugs. He simply walked into this young girl's room, scared the hell out of her, and left her in a state of panic.

"Of course, I refused to take chemo," Rose said. "I was totally hysterical and wanted to leave the hospital that minute. It took my regular doctor and my mother hours to calm me down and convince me to do the treatment."

Rose ultimately spent a year on chemotherapy—while she returned to boarding school.

Dr. William Licamele says that one of the most important aspects of telling the child about the illness is to do so from the child's point of view, to make an effort to think the way the child thinks. For instance, young children do not have a well-developed sense of time. Therefore, telling a 4-year-old that the course of treatment will take "a long time" does not mean much. The next question might be something like, "Will I be okay to go to Billy's birthday party tomorrow?"

Some parents tell their child that he or she is very ill, but they do not use the word *cancer,* they do not mention the possibility of death: "There's something bad in your blood that you have to take medicines to kill." "The lump in your leg has to be cut out, but it has become so large that part of your leg has to be taken off so the bad cells don't have a chance to get loose in other parts of your body."

One mother said, "I had to tell her something about what was going on, and I didn't want to lie to her or minimize how serious things were. But I couldn't use the 'C-word,' and there was no way I could bring myself to say that she might die of this. I suppose if she hadn't gotten better, I would have had to do it. Maybe by then, we all would have gotten used to it somehow. I didn't know then and I still don't know if I did the right thing."

Parents with more than one child tend to provide more details about the illness to all children in the family for several reasons: parents need and expect support and help from the child's siblings; they may know that the siblings will find out about the illness from schoolmates and will "spill the beans" to their sister or brother; and siblings have to be told why their brother or sister is suddenly unable to do certain things. "Why does Lucy have to go to the hospital every afternoon?" is not a question that can be ignored.

Answering questions is never one of the easiest tasks of parenthood, and when the questions are about childhood cancer, it is no wonder that parents often feel paralyzed and have impulses to ignore reality.

The "solution" to the problem is to answer each question as fully as the child needs and wants. The problem, of course, comes in determining what the child needs and wants. When Johnny asks, "Where do I come from?" does he want to know about the birds and the bees, or does he want to know where he was born? If he asks, "Am I going to die?" does he want to know if his life is in jeopardy *that minute* or if the disease will eventually kill him? Does he know what it means to die? Is he really afraid of death, or is he afraid of the disease itself? Or the treatment?

"Answer children's questions slowly," said Leslie Nelson, a clinical social worker in pediatric oncology at Georgetown University Medical Center. "Take it one step at a time and don't give more than one piece of information with each response."

Parents also need to ascertain whether the child understands the answer. "You have a disease called cancer," might mean nothing—or it might conjure up images of the worst possible kind of suffering. Asking the child to repeat the explanation in his or her own words will give parents an idea of how much has been understood. And don't forget that just because the child understands today means that he or she will retain the information tomorrow or next week. As many times as a question is asked, it must be answered.

And parents should not assume that a child's not asking means that he or she understands. "You have to have a little operation to remove the lump" may mean everything or nothing—or anything in between. "Do you remember when we went to visit Grandpa in the hospital?" may or may not be an appropriate association for what the child will experience. It depends on how the child perceived and remembers the visit to grandfather.

Every parent knows that once children enter social relationships with other children, they hear all kinds of things that affect them in a variety of ways. Some are positive and some are not. Children believe the most fantastic stories and they take everything to heart. It is impossible to be fully aware of everything a child knows, thinks, and believes—whether about the characters on *Sesame Street* or about what happened to Billie in the next bed, who left the hospital and was never heard from again.

Coming to grips with the enormity of a child's mind and the possibilities that lie within is daunting. However, children respond to the *way* things are said as much as they do to what is said. Parents who tell their child the bad news with love, hope, patience, and a guarantee of steadfastness of protection will find that the prospect of telling about cancer is not as frightening as it seemed at the outset.

Karen didn't know how dreadfully sick she was. "It wasn't until I was 12 or 13 that I found out what I had. My parents decided not to tell me because they believed that whatever you tell a little kid, they're not going to understand anyway. As I got older, the appropriate time never came to tell me the truth.

"Then when I was 12, we had to transfer our gym records from grammar school to junior high, and I read mine and found out what I had. I read up on it and then told my parents what I knew. We talked about it, and ever since then I've kept up with it [the leukemia], read articles about it, and tried to find out as much as possible. From then on I never let anybody touch me unless they told me exactly what they were going to do."

As time goes on and treatment progresses, parents often add to or change what they told the child originally. Sometimes, too, circumstances change. Either the disease is worse than first believed, or it is not as severe. Perhaps the tumor invaded more normal tissue than the doctors had guessed, and the surgery now will be more extensive than the child had originally been told. Medications are changed in midtreatment and the side effects may be worse or different. Or a course of radiation therapy may not have had the desired effect and might have to be repeated.

Sometimes the child asks for more information or demonstrates that he or she misunderstands things. Dr. Licamele cautions that parents should be certain to find out what the child is asking and what he or she is afraid of. He told the story of a little boy who balked at having his blood drawn for a test. His mother and the lab technician assumed that the child was afraid of the needle (as so many adults are). But what really bothered the little boy was that he thought that *all* his blood was going to be removed. "It was such a simple misunderstanding," said Licamele, "but these things happen all the time. Children ask questions and parents don't take the time to find out what they really want to know."

Sarah wasn't able to tell her son that he had leukemia. The doctors did it for her. "He was in college on the West Coast, and on the Saturday morning after Thanksgiving, he called to tell me he was in the hospital. I was on my way out the door when the phone rang."

Sarah is a medical writer, and when her 20-year-old son described his symptoms and told her how ill he had been—and the fact that his nose had been bleeding for 2 days—she thought immediately of leukemia. "So when the doctor told me he thought that Les had leukemia, I wasn't all that surprised."

But what about the sense of shock? It's one thing to "diagnose" your child who is in a hospital 3,000 miles away, but it's another thing not to be devastated when the news is in fact confirmed.

"I was too busy," Sarah said. "Those first 6 hours were spent gathering information, talking to people, arranging to go to Portland where he was in school, trying to make decisions about how to proceed."

Sarah was forced to bury her fear and shock in a sea of intellectualization and practicality. She didn't know where her husband was, and couldn't locate him until late that afternoon. "By that time, I had already gotten things going, and it was understood that I would be the captain of this effort. We didn't discuss it, but we both knew it."

She was lucky in that she knew many physicians, and she started making phone calls to gather as much data and to get as much advice as possible. "The first decision was whether to treat Les as a child or an adult," she said. "Once that decision was made, we had to decide if it would be appropriate to stabilize him to the point where he could be brought home to Philadelphia."

So it wasn't until she went to bed that night that Sarah was able to let emotional reality creep into her consciousness. And even then, she didn't want to. "I went to bed and told myself that I would think about it tomorrow." Amazingly, she went right to sleep. "But at 1:30 in the morning, my eyes popped open, and that's when it hit me. I couldn't go back to sleep for 2 hours."

When Sarah was asked how she had felt when she walked into her son's hospital room, knowing that he had leukemia, knowing that he knew what he had, she simply closed her eyes as if to shut out the memory. "I felt engulfed in the worst pain you can imagine," was all she could say.

"Going public" with the news—that is, telling co-workers and friends that a child has cancer—evokes all kinds of unpleasant fantasies. Sally's father said, "I dreaded having to tell my boss. Not because he's not a nice guy, but because he would feel sorry for me and in an effort to be helpful, I was afraid he'd tell everyone in the office and they would treat me differently.

"The year before, one of the men who works in another division got AIDS, and everyone went out of their way to be so 'nice' to him that he felt smothered with false affection. One day at lunch, he remarked that sometimes he yearned for the 'bad old days' when he would have been tarred and feathered and then fired in disgrace. He said it as a joke, but it was obviously causing him some pain.

"I didn't want that kind of thing to happen to me, so I put off telling my boss for the longest time, and of course I got obsessed about keeping it a secret, and then I started screwing up on the job, until one day, he called me into his office and asked what was the matter with me.

"I cried again, but by that time, I was so used to my own tears that it didn't bother me as much." The man smiled ruefully as he told the story. "I didn't love crying in front of other people; no one does, but by then I didn't feel as though I was being held up to public ridicule.

"Anyway, after that it was okay. Bernie was terrific about it. I told a few of the people in my own division, but of course it didn't take a week before the whole company knew the story. I just ignored the ones who gushed phony sympathy all over me, and the ones who couldn't deal with it ignored me. So it wasn't as bad as I thought it would be. I guess it hardly ever is."

Getting Expert Help

The initial diagnosis of cancer is usually made by the child's pediatrician, who should refer the family to a pediatric oncologist, if there is one in the area. For people who live where there is no access to specialized pediatric oncology services, which are usually located in a large medical center, a conflict can arise: If the parents want to stay near home, it may have to suffice for the child or adolescent to be treated by an adult oncologist who can be in frequent telephone consultation with colleagues who specialize in childhood cancer. On the other hand, if the parents want the benefit of a sophisticated childhood cancer treatment center, they may have to leave home.

Getting to a specialist as soon as possible is crucial to the child's ultimate recovery because the sooner that effective treatment is instituted, the better the chances of survival. This is true for all types of cancer, but especially so when the disease appears in childhood, because most such cancers attack body cells that grow rapidly. The faster the cancer cells grow, the faster they have to be killed. Chapter 4 explains these concepts in more detail.

If a family is not in a position to find an appropriate means to obtain a second diagnostic opinion, as well as opinions concerning treatment alternatives, there are numerous organizations that can recommend specialists for this purpose (see Appendix A). Even so, the process can be difficult. Often, parents have had to arrange for appropriate specialists themselves and in some cases even fight with the medical system for the best treatment for their child.

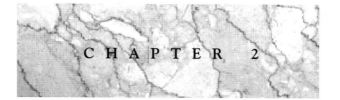

Emotions

Anger

It is entirely normal for parents to be angry, even wildly furious, when their child is diagnosed with cancer. What greater unfairness could life hurl in one's face?

Parents and children are angry at a number of things, many of which they don't recognize. They are especially angry at the disease itself—for causing pain, for frightening them, for stealing a portion of childhood—for its very existence.

Spouses are angry at one another for not being there for each other, for not taking care of the child, for not going to the doctor soon enough, for giving the child a bad genetic endowment.

Children are angry at their parents for not protecting them against this horror. They are angry at their siblings for remaining healthy.

Siblings are angry at the sick child for being sick, for getting all the attention, for making their lives difficult at school and at home.

Parents are angry at children for being sick, for causing so much heartache and anguish, for costing money that the family can't afford.

And everyone is angry at family and friends who don't understand what the parents, child, and siblings are going through, who make uncaring and insensitive remarks, who can't face the fact of the cancer and thus abandon those who need them the most, who do unhelpful things and cast blame.

Anger is everywhere. It comes with the fact of having cancer. The problem is not that the anger exists—we would not be human beings if we did not feel angry at something so unjust. Rather, the problem is coping with our anger, directing it toward useful channels, and letting it escape in appropriate ways.

Naturally, people are not angry all the time, but because anger affects all relationships, strategies for channeling anger in useful ways should be directed toward preventing the opening of old wounds, narrowing whatever rifts exist among family members, and guarding against letting the anger leak out in ways that might be ultimately harmful. Parents describe a variety of techniques they have developed to release anger in ways that cause no harm: playing hard games of high-energy sports; writing down their feelings; and going somewhere where no one can hear them to scream, shout, curse, and otherwise carry on in what most people would consider an unseemly fashion.

Controlled conversations with the targets of anger work if the rules are established in advance (no shouting, no interrupting, no personal attacks, and so forth) and all parties agree to stick to those rules.

Children are scared when they're angry and angry when they're scared. What they are afraid of depends on their age and psychological development. Very young children, for example, are mostly frightened of being separated from their parents, whereas adolescents fear damage to their physical selves and changes in the way they look.

All children—all people—hate pain and discomfort, but if they can name the fear and anger and act out their feelings, the negative emotions are not as overpowering.

Art therapy or play therapy can help children deal with anger. They can use crayons and paints to draw the "big bad cancer," they can use color to express feelings, and they can act out feelings in plays, skits, and dances. They can also personify feelings with dolls and puppets.

Bill, who was a teenager when he got cancer, was asked where he turned when things got really dark and when the anger threatened to go out of control.

"I turned to Demerol, I turned to Valium, and I turned to marijuana. I slept to escape and withdraw."

The marijuana eased his nausea and enhanced the effects of the analgesics, so he used to go off in his wheelchair far away from his room and the other patients, look out the window, and smoke.

During the course of his treatment, he said that he "went out on the street a lot" to be with his friends, but his appearance (pale, thin, hairless, and sickly) "freaked people out." It was hard for Bill to describe exactly what he meant, but it was clear that people's reactions to his appearance and illness caused him a great deal of pain.

Bill has recovered now, and although he is not completely happy, he is working full-time and no longer smokes marijuana or takes other drugs.

Arthur, on the other hand, controlled his grief and anger by controlling his fear. When asked whether he had thought he would die, he said, "I thought I might, but you can't go on living thinking you're going to die. I never really thought about dying. I looked at it like an obstacle. If I could overcome that [the cancer], there's no telling what I could do. Now I feel that, within limits, I can survive anything. I feel stronger. I think determination and a positive attitude helped me to pull through. I always had the feeling that I was going to beat it, that I was going to come out of it, and that I'd be a better person afterward."

Arthur said that being so sick taught him to appreciate the "little" things: moving about without having his arms restrained by intravenous tubes and getting out of bed and looking at the sky. "What I learned the most is not to take anything for granted," he said. "Just being able to move freely when I sleep and wake up and walk around. That's the lesson I learned."

Bobby's cancer was diagnosed when he was 14, and now he thinks of himself as an adult—"adult-minded, that is."

He said it has little to do with having had cancer, and maybe in a way he's right. Perhaps any catastrophe would have pushed him along the road to adulthood faster than his contemporaries.

His home life probably had much to do with his growing up fast. He "learned a lot" from having cancer. "I can take a lot of pain and pressure without thinking anything of it."

This last is probably bravado. He *has* endured great pain, but it preys on his mind more than he is willing to admit. For example, when asked if there were times when he thought he was going to die, he said there were, but the Lord helped him through. His smile was a little shaky, though.

He talked about two other patients he got to know in the hospital and how he felt when they died. Why did he think he survived when they didn't?

He shrugged. "I don't know. Maybe it's because I'm special. For some reason the Lord is telling me to start my life early." Bobby is not sure just what "special" means, but he is certain that the word applies to him. God chose *him* to survive.

Bobby used the expression "to start my life" to mean living as an adult—on his own, out from under his family's thumb. He said it often, as if what he is experiencing—the cancer, the emotional deprivation, and the verbal and physical abuse of which he had been a victim at home—isn't his real life. He discounts the present as not "real" so it won't hurt as much. He said that he always feels "in a rush."

"Maybe the Lord is telling me to rush because I'm not going to live long. Maybe that's why he wants me to start my life early."

Denial

Denial is a powerful emotional tool that often can be used to good advantage. However, it also can prevent parents from obtaining immediate help for a child, or compel an adolescent to refuse treatment.

Parents use a wide variety of denial mechanisms to protect themselves from the pain and fear of knowing that their child has cancer. Some intellectualize the illness and collect vast amounts of medical information on the subject. Some even carry this technique to an almost pernicious end by believing that they can manage their child's treatment better than physicians.

Intellectualization is a way to deny feelings and manage stress, and can be used positively or negatively. Learning everything that it is possible for a layperson to understand about childhood cancer and the treatment is one way to increase control over a situation in which control is slipping away at an alarming rate.

Children often make their cancer a subject of school reports, probably in an effort to explain to teachers and classmates what's wrong with them without having to personalize the experience more than is comfortable.

Some parents turn to religion for strength in the face of what they perceive as overwhelming disaster. Sometimes too much "responsibility" is placed in the hands of God and the child is denied appropriate treatment. Still others never accept the diagnosis and trudge from one doctor to another seeking false hope, thereby denying their child the advantage of immediate treatment.

Using denial as a psychological technique can have benefits as well. Denying feelings of hopelessness can force parents back on the track of practicality and help them attend to the parts of their lives that they may have ignored in the face of overwhelming grief. It can also lessen the preoccupation with the disease, and it can minimize the terror that many parents say accompanies their every waking hour. It can be especially useful when the direct result of denial is positive action.

The reaction that is precisely the opposite of denial is premature despair—that is, caving in immediately upon hearing the diagnosis and assuming that death will be inevitable. A physician at Johns Hopkins Hospital in Baltimore described an adolescent who was told bluntly that she had leukemia and was taken to a mortuary to select her own casket and make funeral arrangements—all while she was still in relatively good health.

Victor used denial to get through most of his treatment. He was 13 when he was diagnosed with Hodgkin's disease. "I said [to myself], 'this is a bad cold. I'll do whatever I have to do to get through it.'"

He never thought of himself as seriously ill, even though his treatment consisted of radiation and chemotherapy—not exactly appropriate for a common cold, even a bad one. He spent 20 days in Memorial Sloan-Kettering Cancer Center, but no one ever said the "C-word" to him, and he never used it when thinking about his illness. He is 32 years old now and still shies away from the dread word.

During his time as an inpatient, Victor never left his room except when he was taken elsewhere for treatment. Even as long ago as 1974, when he was diagnosed, Memorial Sloan-Kettering had sophisticated ancillary treatment for children. There were social workers, play rooms, play therapy—all the accoutrements for helping children cope with the crisis. Victor refused them all. "I stayed in my room and read and played war games and watched television. No one but my parents was allowed to visit."

Not his sister, not his grandparents, not his school friends. No one. Victor succeeded in isolating himself almost totally. One has the impression that the only reason his parents visited Victor in the hospital was that he had no choice but to allow it.

What did he think about all that time? Why did he think he was in a cancer center? What did he feel when he saw other children with cancer? Was he afraid? Did he think of death? How did he cope?

The surprising answer is that Victor did not think about it—beyond believing that he had a "bad cold." He refused to be scared, because what's so frightening about a cold? He didn't entertain the possibility that he might die because he wasn't that sick in the first place. The seriousness of his situation never became a reality for Victor.

How did this young man manage to "fall into" a state of denial so quickly and so expertly when faced with the news that he had what he must have known, on some level, was a life-threatening illness?

He said he doesn't know, but it seems that he must have been "practicing" for many years. Perhaps he had always responded to any unpleasantness that crossed his path by denying its existence or its effect on him.

Carrying denial to this extent is a "neat trick," but it has serious disadvantages. Victor is now carrying around emotional baggage that he doesn't know he has. Although he is a friendly, intelligent, and outgoing person, it takes a stranger only a few minutes to bump up against the wall of defenses that Victor has erected to protect himself, not only from the fear of recurrence, but from any emotional openness. He is a closed-off person who has trouble developing and maintaining intimate relationships.

It is also tempting to surmise that Victor's upbeat, cheerful demeanor hides a powerful depression that may someday come crashing through these barriers, which may not be as strong as he hopes.

Grief

It is a common reaction when thinking about grief to think about death—that is, about someone having died. But people grieve about things other than the loss of someone loved. In childhood cancer, the grief is for the loss of the way things were. "Nothing will ever be the same again" is a phrase that one hears over and over.

The feeling of loss that accompanies childhood cancer is different from, but no less acute than, the grief that arises from death. It is the loss of years of carefree and unfettered physical well-being; loss of a limb or other body part; loss of simplicity in relationships, perhaps even the loss of friends; loss of independence for a time; loss of the ability to think of oneself in a certain way, as physically whole, for example; and, perhaps most important, the loss of innocence.

Farther along in the treatment, children grieve over the death of other children with cancer. These children—who meet in the hospital, in the clinic, and in support groups and camps—make friends with one another very quickly and form close attachments. When one of them dies, the fear in each child comes rushing to the surface. "If Linda and I had the same diagnosis, and she died after having gotten the same kind of treatment, that means I could die too."

It is rare for parents to be experienced in helping children cope with the death of someone their own age. And when another child dies of cancer, parents are as horrified as their children—and as frightened. It would be easy to deny the fear ("Linda died, but you're not going to"), but that is a mistake. The death of a "cancer colleague" has to be talked about and cried over in the same way that all other aspects of the illness have to be talked about and cried over.

Depression

When anger and grief are directed inward, they can turn into energy-sapping depression. Not only is this not helpful, it can be debilitating. Parents need all the strength they can muster to make arrangements for their child's treatment, as well as to attend to their other children and continue to earn a living.

Sarah described it as a sense of powerlessness, of being out of control. "You can't imagine that your child would get so sick and that there would be nothing you could do about it," she said. "Always before, whatever the problem, you took your kid to the doctor if that's what was necessary, or you washed the cut and put on a Band-Aid and gave him a cookie. You could always kiss it and make it better. You're never pre-pared for the *hugeness* of cancer, the way it just takes over your life.

"Everything else just falls away," she added. "There is nothing in your life but the cancer and the fact that your child might die. It's totally consuming."

This is one way that people perceive depression, which has a variety of external and internal symptoms: sadness, crying unexpectedly and for no apparent reason, irritability, insomnia, decreased appetite (or com-pulsive eating), restlessness, boredom, diminished sex drive, lack of in-terest in appearance, and diminished physical energy—sometimes to such an extent that a person ceases to function.

But most parents do not allow themselves to get to that point be-cause they *cannot* allow it—because their child needs and depends on them. Many parents who are depressed find themselves stuck within feelings of gloom and seemingly perpetual bad weather. Sarah said, "No matter how nice a day it was, it always seemed to be raining on *me*!"

There are ways to combat these feelings:

- Dress in bright, cheerful colors. *Do* get dressed every day.
- Have plenty of green plants and fresh flowers around. Tend your garden. Surround your child with plants and flowers. Living things are reminders of continuing life.
- Get out of the house at least once a day for a pleasurable activity of even the simplest kind.
- Exercise every day. A long walk with a dog (yours or a neighbor's) is calming.
- Stay in the light as much as possible, especially in winter. Go out-doors on sunny days and keep the indoor environment well lit.
- Structure your day so you don't have huge blocks of time with noth-ing to do. Depression characteristically feeds on itself; keeping your

mind occupied with external activities prevents you from dwelling on depressing thoughts. If necessary, write your activities down on an hour-by-hour basis so there's always a goal to be accomplished.

- Plan activities in advance—preferably with other people, so that you are obligated to do them.
- Spend time with healthy children—your own and others.
- Always bring a book or something to engage your mind while waiting at the clinic for your child. Or use that waiting time to exercise or run errands.

Jacqueline's mother said, "The first time I heard myself laugh after she got sick, I looked around in amazement to see who it was. How could I be enjoying myself so much when she was upstairs recovering from a particularly difficult bout of chemotherapy?"

This mother felt guilty for having a good time while her daughter was so sick, and the first hint that life could be enjoyable, even in the face of pain that had at first seemed unbearable, created all sorts of feelings that she wasn't prepared to deal with at the time.

She did, however, talk about the experience in her mothers' support group and heard how another woman had burst into tears in the dressing room of a department store as she looked in the mirror and took pleasure in a new dress. "My son had lost so much weight that his pants were always in danger of falling down, and his hair had fallen out in clumps so that he looked like a space alien," the mother said. "But I looked great in that royal blue dress, and the guilt for liking my appearance while Terry looked so ghastly almost knocked me over."

Aftermath of the Diagnosis

Cancer is probably one of the most feared words in any language. It is a metaphor for evil.

Fear of cancer is real and rational, but it can be tamed by understanding the disease—how its various types differ from one another, how the body reacts to the presence of the invasive cancer cells, and how those cells are affected by treatment.

Generally, the more control one has over a situation, the less there is to fear. In childhood cancer, if parents—and the child—are given some responsibility for, and thus control over, the treatment, they will understand more and be less afraid. All family members, including the sick child and siblings, need to know what is happening, what progress is being made, and what problems must be faced. Everyone needs to be alone sometimes to think about things or to cry or to just lie on their back and think of nothing. Too much privacy and isolation, however, can lead to loneliness (even in a houseful of people) and the tendency to dwell on the negative aspects of what has befallen the family. As one mother said, "Some of the dramas I wrote in my mind could have rivaled Shakespeare for pure tragedy."

Childhood cancer is terribly disruptive to families, but it need not mean unmitigated gloom. Sometimes the stress and tension seem unbearable, and sometimes harsh words are spoken. Tempers fray. But there are also times of intense closeness, of a drawing together and a desire to hold and comfort that were not present before. In fact, some families report that their lives have improved and that solving the problems of how to get through the crisis has brought them closer together and had a positive effect on all their relationships. When the family receives good counseling and support, these times can be more frequent than the flashes of anger and the hurtful release of tension.

Ian's mother went through an emotional and logistical nightmare when her 3-year-old child got sick—and she had to do it alone. "My husband was stationed at a small naval base in Italy at the time. I kept taking Ian to the base doctor because I knew there was something definitely wrong with him. They thought it was hookworm because it was so common in Italian children.

"By the time it occurred to the doctors to do a blood test—and they did it only because I screamed and yelled and forced them to—Ian was really sick. He had a hemoglobin of only 4—way below normal."

Ian and his mother were put on a plane for Weisbaden, West Germany, so he could be evaluated at the large naval hospital there. "I had only time to get a change of clothes and to pack a few things for Ian before we left. My husband was put on emergency leave, but he had the other kids to look after, so I was on my own."

Pat was told only that Ian had a very severe case of "pernicious anemia," but she is a smart woman who responds well to nonverbal cues, so she knew that it was something far worse. But she learned of her youngest child's diagnosis in one of the coldest, most insensitive ways imaginable: "When the plane landed, everyone seemed to know where they were going, or people met them. We weren't told anything and were standing alone on the tarmac—me dressed for Italian weather, and Ian in nothing more than his PJs and bathrobe. I was trying to decide what to do when this corpsman ran up and said, 'Is this the kid who's dying of leukemia?' "

Christine was 14 years old and living with her mother and brother in a Washington, D.C. ghetto when her cancer was diagnosed. She thought she would surely die of the disease, because at the time she had never heard of anyone surviving it. "I'm very scared of death—very scared."

How did she learn to cope with the fear?

"My mother was a great help, and so were all the nurses on the floor.

They treated me as part of their family. They were really nice. They comforted me when the treatment was bad, and they pushed me to keep on going. They really helped."

She said that understanding the disease and the treatment also helped, as did meeting people who had responded well to treatment. Gradually she came to believe she would not die. "If they can do it, I can do it," she said. "I saw a little girl who had pulled through. She was so small and here she was surviving. Then I began to see a whole lot of people on that floor and coming to the hematology clinic who had cancer and were surviving. It strikes all ages and all colors, and I began to see that my cancer wasn't as severe as some other people's. That helped a whole lot."

Christine progressed from fear, despair, and a potentially life-threatening illness to hope, a positive attitude, and good health. This is typical of children who survive cancer.

But she is unique in that she—and others like her—came out on the other side of the disease in her own way. Yes, she had the help of her mother and the entire pediatric oncology team at the hospital, but her survival was her own.

Hospital social workers and other therapists can help families deal with feelings and reactions. Anne Dente described the effects of a diagnosis of childhood cancer on the way families function: "Most stay together and weather the storm, but some that had been on the verge of breaking up crack under the strain."

It is not necessarily true, she said, that the mother always carries the lion's share of the emotional burden. "We see many nurturing, caretaking fathers. Sometimes it's cultural or ethnic, but we see such a wide variety of people that it's impossible to predict how mothers and fathers will react."

Disciplining a Child With Cancer

Most professionals recommend that discipline be maintained for the sick child. It might appear almost cruel to punish a child who is so seriously ill, and it seems natural to let the child do and have whatever he or she desires.

This is a mistake.

Withdrawing discipline is jarring, and the child may misinterpret it. For instance, if the parents have been honest about the seriousness of the illness while still hopeful about the chances for recovery, the child could think, "They *say* I'm going to get better, but they're letting me do all the things I was never allowed to do before. That must mean that they feel *really* sorry for me, and maybe I *am* going to die. Why else would they be so lenient?"

This is scary.

Maintaining discipline and established limits demonstrates love and caring, and even a hint of withdrawal of love at so crucial a time could be devastating.

Withdrawal of discipline can signal withdrawal of hope—for both parents and child. In other words, the way children are disciplined reflects, to a great extent, the family's values and their sense of place in the world. Discipline is a way of teaching children which behaviors are acceptable and which ones are not. It is a way of inculcating socially and professionally appropriate behavior: "If you understand the reasons for picking up your toys when you're finished playing and for hanging up your clothes when you take them off, and if you get in the habit of doing that, you'll be more likely to hand in your school assignments on time and to type them neatly."

Firm and consistent discipline is also a way of teaching respect for others: "Don't interrupt your mother while she's speaking, and you will learn to listen to what others have to say."

Setting limits and establishing good habits are preparation for the future. If these are ignored, a child with cancer could easily come to believe that he or she *has* no future.

This is unfair.

It also has the potential for creating unnecessary conflict among siblings, which can lead to chaos in the household. "Jimmy doesn't have to wipe up the milk *he* spilled, so I don't see why I have to do it either. It's not fair!"

Jimmy's little sister is correct: It isn't fair. It isn't fair that her brother got cancer, but there is nothing that parents can do about that. Parents *can*, however, do something about preventing imbalances of justice in the household. Even when control over the medical situation seems minimal at best, meting out discipline and punishment in equal measure among siblings is one sphere over which parents can maintain control.

If parents relax discipline for the sick child out of a sense of their own guilt and powerlessness, a burden is placed on the child, who doesn't deserve it and probably cannot cope with it. A parent's unconscious thought process might go something like this: "If only I had done such-and-such or not done this or that, Susie wouldn't be sick now. Somehow it's my fault, so in order to make up for what I did—or what I didn't do—I'll let her behave however she wants. She can have as much ice cream as she can eat, and I won't punish her when she breaks the rules. It's the least I can do."

This is dangerous.

It's a treacherous road to travel because such thoughts multiply. As the child's behavior worsens, the parents' guilt increases, and the situation soon turns unmanageable. The child turns into a "holy terror," and parents' tempers begin to fray—and eventually snap.

The same theory holds true for household chores and responsibilities. The sick child should be expected to do as much as he or she can. This means that if taking the garbage cans to the curb was always Leonard's job, it still should be Leonard's job as long as he can manage it. If one big plastic can is too heavy, then an arrangement should be made to make the chore easier: buy a can on wheels or teach him to take the can to the curb empty and make several trips with smaller loads to fill it.

The point is that Leonard may ultimately have to live and work with some type of disability, and the sooner he learns to adapt to it, the happier he will be. Even if he will eventually recover all his strength and health, he ought to be taught that his role in the family and in the larger community does not diminish because he has had a physical illness. Leonard's responsibility *to* others is not negated by the fact that he has been ill and has received obligations *from* others.

Learning to live happily and productively in society is a task achieved step by step over the course of a lifetime. The most fundamental lessons are learned early and they are learned in the home. For a parent to waive those lessons because a child has cancer is to handicap him or her in far-reaching ways that have nothing to do with the physical illness.

Factors That Influence the Way Families React

A variety of personal and socioeconomic factors affect the ways families experience and react to childhood cancer.

Child's Age at Diagnosis

According to Chesler and Barbarin (1987), parents experience greater stress when the child is more than 7 years old at the time of diagnosis. First, it seems more difficult to explain the fact of cancer—and the possibility of death—to an older child, even though he or she may have an easier time grasping the concepts intellectually. Perhaps it is *because* the child can understand the seriousness of what is happening that the parents feel such pain.

Then, too, children diagnosed at a later age are already out in the world and have their own lives. They no longer "belong" exclusively to their parents, who cannot totally shield and protect them. The lives of children who are in school, who are on junior soccer teams, who have parts in plays, and who belong to Girl Scout troops are far more disrupted than those who have not yet graduated from their strollers. Older children worry about things and are sophisticated enough to put names to those worries. They understand what the future could bring.

Family Status

Contrary to what one might expect, some single parents experience less social and personal stress than coupled parents. Single parents have developed extremely workable coping skills and are confident in their ability to handle things. It is true that they do not have the emotional and practical support of a spouse, but neither do they have to devote energy to maintaining a spousal relationship. They can, therefore, devote themselves totally to the sick child. Other children of single parents are used to helping with household tasks and taking more responsibility for their own lives and will probably be more likely to take on the added burdens imposed by the illness without too much complaint. Chapter 8 discusses this issue in more detail.

It is a myth that marriages tend to fall apart under the stress of childhood cancer—unless they were on the verge of breaking up anyway. Strong, healthy marriages usually improve as the family adjusts to the fact of cancer, but weak marriages can be torn further asunder by the stress.

Money and Logistics

Distance from the hospital has a tremendous effect on stress levels for two reasons. First are the obvious logistical and financial problems, which exact tremendous wear and tear. Second is the psychological stress: The further away from home one has to go for medical treatment, the bigger, grander, and more frightening the hospital seems—and the greater the fear that the illness must be especially serious and complex. This may not be true at all, especially for people who live in areas where there is no medical care to speak of, but if it *seems* that way, then a frightened mind says that it *is* that way.

Even when the cancer is in permanent remission and the long trips for treatment are over, parents (and older children) worry that a sudden relapse will place them in serious jeopardy if they are far from the doctors and nurses who have become familiar to them.

Being away from home, friends, and family also tends to increase stress. Ian was a "Navy brat" when his leukemia was diagnosed, but the fabled closeness and camaraderie of military life did not seem to work for his mother. On the contrary, she encountered practically every snafu that military life is famous for.

"After he was diagnosed in Weisbaden, we were flown immediately to the Bethesda Naval Hospital. I had $63 in cash with me, only two or three changes of clothes, and absolutely no idea of what was going to happen once we got to Bethesda."

Ian was admitted to the pediatric unit right away, but it was a Saturday and no one seemed to care what happened to his mother. The hospital had a lodge where patients' families could stay if they had no other option, but it was full, and no one offered to help Pat find a place to stay. "I didn't even have enough money to get a motel room for the night, and although I called my two children who were in college, it would take them a while to get to me.

"My husband could get emergency leave, but there was some sort of communications mix-up and he never was notified, so I didn't see him for almost 3 weeks."

Pat was devastated by fear, grief, and loneliness. She was positive that Ian was going to die. "I was all alone and had no place to stay, no one to talk to—I didn't know what I was going to do."

Although she refused to allow herself the luxury of tears, she did vent her anger to the people who managed the lodge. When a woman passing through the lobby overheard Pat's tale of woe, she offered to share her room, and Pat stayed with her for several days.

Finances have an obvious effect on stress levels. Chapter 11 discusses paying for treatment in detail. Suffice it to say here that a family that has no health insurance, or inadequate coverage, can be financially wiped out in a few weeks when a child develops cancer. In addition, poor people tend to have fewer resources and less access to information than do people with more money.

Environment

Sarah said that her physical surroundings had a lot to do with the amount of stress she experienced and the way she handled it. "When Les first got sick and we flew out to Portland, I had the sense that the hospital out there did everything they could to provide ease and comfort for the families."

She described two beautifully furnished rooms that were set aside for the exclusive use of families of cancer patients. One had a small kitchen with coffee, tea, condiments, crackers, dishes, and plastic cutlery. There was a television set that wasn't turned on all the time and an AM-FM radio. The other room was like a meditation chapel, also with comfortable chairs. It had dim lighting, no television, no radio—and a few religious artifacts here and there. "You could go in there and just be quiet," said Sarah. "If people talked, they did it in whispers, but mostly there was silence."

The nurses encouraged families to bring food to patients, and there was a 24-hour-a-day snack shop that made the kind of milkshakes that Les liked. Families were allowed, even encouraged, to visit patients whenever they liked.

"But when we brought him back to Philadelphia, it was just the opposite. The hospital had this big, fancy medical reputation, but the whole place was run specifically to meet the needs of the staff. Hardly anyone was nice to us, and no one even bothered to answer our questions unless I made a big stink about it."

Sarah described the one room set aside for families. "It was small and incredibly filthy with these ugly plastic chairs. Visiting hours were over at 8:00 in the evening, and again, I had to make a lot of noise just so my husband and I could take turns sitting with Les while he watched TV.

"It felt like the patients were there for the benefit of the staff, not the other way around. And the families—well, we felt as if we were more of a nuisance than anything else."

Children's Reactions

Children grieve too, and are afraid. They feel guilty and blame themselves for getting sick. Depending on how old they are and what they understand about the illness, they can work through their feelings with loving help. They go through a bad time and then recover.

The way children react to learning that they have cancer depends on a number of factors: their self-concept and self-esteem; their place within the family and the way they interact with other members; how they function at school; the length and complexity of the proposed treatment; the site of the tumor (which has a great deal to do with the visibility of the cancer and the likelihood of permanent physical impairment); their emotional and intellectual development; the way their parents react to the news; the manner in which they are told; and the responses and attitudes of their peers and others in the community.

Needs Vary According to Age

Infancy

Infancy represents absolute purity, hope, total goodness, and an unblemished spirit. Therefore, when such a tiny creature is struck with cancer, the tragedy seems all the more cruel.

In fact, the opposite is probably true. If a child is fated to have cancer, early is "better" than later because a child who develops cancer at less than 1 year of age generally has a better prognosis than an older child. The tumors (with the exception of brain tumors) are less malignant. In addition, with the exception of radiation which can have severe dose- and age-related toxic effects in infants, babies under a year old have a much higher tolerance for treatment than do older children.

One of the major problems with cancer in little babies is that many of the symptoms mimic other far more benign childhood health problems: changes in eating and elimination, behavioral changes, fever, and general irritability. If these symptoms are sufficiently severe for the baby to be taken to the doctor, most pediatricians do not immediately think of cancer unless they find a particularly large tumor.

In addition, a baby can't tell its parents what is wrong. Although this may seem like a frivolous and disrespectful comparison, many young parents who have had years of experience with pets are accustomed to be on the lookout for nonverbal signs of health problems. A dog that loses its appetite or a cat that suddenly stops washing itself is telling its owner that something is seriously wrong. A baby who has diarrhea for more than a day or who begins to spit up all her formula is telling her parents the same thing.

Contrary to what one might expect, and perhaps contrary to our emotional reactions, surgery in an infant is almost never contraindicated. Babies tolerate surgery very well.

Cancer in infancy has some unique characteristics:

ᵃ Neuroblastoma is the most common cancer during the first year of life, followed by retinoblastoma, hepatoblastoma, and Wilms' tumor.

ᵃ Neuroblastoma is almost always curable if the diagnosis is made early and if tumor cells do not metastasize to the liver.

ᵃ Wilms' tumor has its highest frequency immediately after birth; its incidence decreases sharply after 3 months of age.

ᵃ Hodgkin's disease affects boys three times more often than girls.

ᵃ Ewing's sarcoma is almost never seen in nonwhites.

ᵃ Age is an important factor in the prognosis of acute lymphoblastic (or lymphocytic) leukemia (ALL).

ᵃ Kidney tumors (mesoblastic nephromas) are often congenital—that is, a baby is born with the disease.

Parents of small babies with cancer tend to react somewhat differently than the parents of older children. Infants, especially those under 3 months of age, are viewed as not quite separate individuals, not yet persons in their own right. Therefore, a mother might "take on" her baby's diagnosis as her own and see herself as sick.

Many mothers blame themselves and associate the cancer with events during pregnancy: what they ate or did not eat, what they drank, the cigarettes they smoked, the sonograms they had, the medications they took—even what they thought about while they were pregnant. Some mothers are unfortunate enough to have blame—real or implied—heaped on them by husbands, parents, and in-laws.

On the other side of the coin, some parents blame obstetricians and initiate unjustified lawsuits because they don't know where to direct their anger. Everyone wants a perfect baby, and many of the reactions that parents have when their child is born with a birth defect are the same as parents have when their infant develops cancer. They mourn the loss of perfection, they agonize over the suffering of an innocent creature, they grieve over the presence of sickroom supplies in a nursery, they feel frustration about not being to explain or ease the suffering, they anguish over separation from their new child, they cry in loneliness, they worry about the fragility of a new infant, and they're certain they won't be able to care for their baby at home.

And they fear death.

Parents of a hospitalized baby should be allowed as much contact with the child as possible. The following are some ways that parents can help their infant—and themselves—get through the experience:

- Feed, dress, hold, and cuddle the baby as you would at home. Most hospitals are very cooperative about allowing parents to visit whenever they want, at any time of the day or night, but if the hospital balks at what it sees as "inconvenient" visiting, you should insist that you be allowed full access to your baby.
- Bring the baby's clothes, blankets, toys, and stuffed animals to the hospital.
- Participate in your baby's treatment as much as possible. Learn how to give medications (by mouth and by injection), how to change dressings, and how to do whatever else the baby needs. The more hands-on care an infant receives from its own parents rather than hospital staff, the less traumatic the experience will be.
- Make certain that siblings and grandparents visit the baby as often as they wish.
- Make audio and video tapes of yourselves and other immediate family members to play for the baby when you cannot be there. Talk a lot on the tape, sing songs, and play with the child's toys.

Early Childhood

Children younger than 5 or 6 years of age probably cannot understand the seriousness of what is wrong with them. They certainly cannot grasp the idea of death as a permanent state.

Nevertheless, children have to be told something, and should be told the truth. What a child can understand about the illness is related to his or her age and level of sophistication. But whatever the child's cognitive ability, the news should be broken in stages, escalating slowly. For example, "There's a lump in your tummy" may not be especially threatening, particularly if the parent talks about it and touches the lump in a friendly, caressing way. Moreover, the child probably has noticed the lump already and may or may not have thought that it was anything out of the ordinary.

The next stage might be, "The lump is not a friendly lump [or a good lump], and the doctor wants to take it away because it's not good for little children to have tummy lumps."

This still probably will not be especially frightening. It is only when the subjects of hospitalization and surgery are introduced that the child will know that there is something really wrong.

Hospitalization presents its own problems for very young children. Their fear is less of the nature of the illness (for they cannot comprehend its gravity) than of separation from their parents and the implicit threat of abandonment.

Children under the age of 10 often perceive illness as punishment. Very little ones blame outside forces ("That nasty hose made me trip and fall"), but when they get a little older, they tend to blame themselves, especially for having bad thoughts ("I wished my sister dead, and now I'm being punished").

It is crucial at this point that parents shower their children with love and the reassurance that they will not be abandoned, that the illness and hospitalization are in no way their fault, that they are not being punished for the mischief they got into last week—or even for their mischievous thoughts.

One of the worst parts of the whole experience—the thing that parents hate almost the most—is that their child must be subjected to a variety of frightening and painful medical tests. Parents can remain with the child for some of the tests (needle sticks, even spinal taps), but for others, they have no choice but to wait alone and worry.

Such situations are always traumatic for both parent and child. There is no way to anticipate what a young child will think or feel, and there is no way to completely banish fear. There are, however, techniques for making a terrifying situation less so:

ᴥ Children fear the unknown and unfamiliar. Therefore, if possible, take the child to visit the hospital before admission. This will create some sense of familiarity, although nothing looks the same from a stretcher or wheelchair as it does from an upright position holding mommy's hand.

- During the preadmission visit, or after admission but before the tests begin, take the child to visit some of the high-tech areas where he or she will be treated. This is especially important for places where the equipment is large and might appear menacing—for example, the X-ray department or the operating suite.
- Have the child meet as many of the hospital personnel as possible before admission. This will provide some sense of mastery and control.
- If possible, introduce the child to others of his or her age who have cancer. This is more helpful when the child is older—that is, at least 4 or 5 years old.
- Make certain that the hospitalized child plays with other patients as much and as often as practical. Play is vital.
- Role-play what is going to happen in the hospital. Many pediatric oncology centers have child life therapists who can help with this activity and offer suggestions.
- Use a series of incentives and rewards for enduring difficult or painful tests and procedures. These should not be rewards for "being good" or not crying; rather, they are simply "congratulations" for getting through the ordeal—in *any* emotional shape.
- Use distractions such as emotive imagery (how a favorite cartoon hero would cope with the situation, for instance), hypnosis, video games, fantasy play, music via earphones, and the like during procedures. These distractions can be highly effective in reducing pain and anxiety.
- If you cannot accompany your child during a procedure, tell him or her exactly where you will be when it is over—and then *be there* with hugs and kisses and a reward.
- Tell the truth about what will happen during a test or procedure. If it will hurt, say so. Do not emphasize the pain, but don't lie about it.
- Tell the truth about the consequences of treatment. This is terribly difficult, and any parent would rather do almost anything than tell a child that his or her leg must be amputated or that hair will begin to fall out in clumps (a young child will have no sense of the future when hair will grow back in). However, it is not a task that parents can shirk and still retain their child's complete trust.

❧ Stay with the child as much as possible. During the first few days, either the mother or the father (or a grandparent who knows the child well) should be with the child at all times, including all night long. Most pediatric oncology units have comfortable reclining chairs for adults in the children's rooms; however, if one is not available, you will have to be uncomfortable for a few nights. As the child gets used to the hospital and his or her fear recedes, you can begin to taper off the all-night vigils.

❧ Children often are frightened when they believe their parents are helpless to do anything for them. Therefore, it is helpful for you to participate as much as you can in giving them physical care: bathing, changing beds, helping them dress, giving medications, and so forth.

Middle Childhood

School-age children face many of the same fears as little ones, but because they know and understand more, they are even more concerned about threats to their bodily integrity. Many of them respond to the news of their illness with psychosomatic complaints (a headache or stomachache—something more familiar). They have nightmares; their emotions and moods change rapidly and with no apparent outside stimulus. Sometimes they regress into babyhood and sometimes they demonstrate "adult" acceptance.

Parents should not be fooled by this last reaction. Johnny is not "taking it like a man." He is scared silly, but he probably believes that his parents want him to act grown up—and so he tries. However, his fear will eventually leak out in other ways. It is better to deal with it at the outset.

School-age children can be very verbal, and they want to know details. As parents have already found out, children of this age ask questions about everything, and this characteristic does not disappear when the subject at hand is cancer. Many of their questions are poignantly difficult, but children take great pride in learning things, especially in knowing the correct medical terminology for their illness and all the treatments.

In families that are not used to open communication, this curiosity will be difficult to handle, and it may be a good idea for the child to spend time alone with his or her physician discussing the illness and treatment. This will take some of the responsibility off the parents' shoulders and will make the child feel mature, as if he or she also has a role to play in managing the cancer.

Some children withdraw and become more and more dependent on one parent, usually the mother. It would be easy to encourage this behavior, to create a private dyad that excludes the other parent, the siblings—even the rest of the world. This is not a good idea, however. Children of this age need to continue the group activities that are so much a part of their lives. They need to play with one another, and they need to develop the motor and social skills that are crucial to middle childhood.

Adolescence

Adolescents present a unique set of problems. The term *childhood cancer* is difficult because teenagers do not see themselves as children. They have begun the struggle for independence and greatly resent the return to a more dependent position forced by the illness.

Young people worry about the illness itself and about becoming a burden on their family, but often they hesitate to share these concerns. Not having an outlet for such thoughts can lead to isolation, loneliness, and depression.

Adolescents are concerned about their appearance and acceptance by peers (and sometimes resent their healthy friends), about their burgeoning sexuality, and about their schooling and future. All of these areas are threatened by the cancer. Resentment at being placed in a sick role runs high and many adolescents have a hard time adjusting to it, especially those who had always been very physically active.

This is also the time when young people begin to take a greater interest in the world around them and to seriously consider their place in the grand scheme of things. They start to develop mature religious and spiritual beliefs, which can be severely tested by the cancer. Like their parents, some come out of the experience with a stronger belief in God, and some lose whatever budding faith they had.

They all ask, "Why me?"

Joan was 16 when she got ALL. "I had a bad cold that wouldn't go away," she said, "but my mother didn't worry until a big lymph node popped out on my neck. Even then, we didn't think it was much of anything because my sister had had something like that just a few months before, and it turned out to be nothing."

Joan's major concern was that she had mononucleosis and would have to miss the rest of the school year. Her family pediatrician sent her to a specialist ("I didn't know what an oncologist was, so even that didn't scare me"), who took one look at her and said, "I think you have some form of Hodgkin's disease."

"And then he just walked out of the room and left my mother and me there alone. She started to cry because she knew what Hodgkin's was, and that was when I first got scared."

Within 2 hours, Joan was on an operating table at the local community hospital for a biopsy of the lymph node. Three days after that, she was transferred to the pediatric oncology unit at Johns Hopkins Hospital in Baltimore, about an hour's drive from home.

"The difference was like night and day," she said. "The people at Anne Arundel [the local hospital] were okay, but they didn't have any idea of how to talk to a 16-year-old who had just been diagnosed with ALL."

So they ignored her. "The nurses did what they had to do, but they treated me like a lump in the bed. When I got to Hopkins, it was a whole different story. They said, 'Okay, you have leukemia. This is what we're going to do.' They treated it very matter-of-factly, and everyone was very positive. They just assumed that I would get better."

Johns Hopkins has a young adult unit, but Joan was placed on the pediatric ward. That had advantages and disadvantages. "All the other patients were no older than 6 or 7, so I didn't have anyone my own age to talk to. But on the other hand, the nurses and social workers and everyone else were really nice. They were used to dealing with kids who had cancer so they could put me at ease. They all had this real upbeat attitude."

Joan's boyfriend came to visit her every evening, and classmates she barely knew visited her or sent cards or notes.

But Joan's best friend never spoke to her again. "Once she found out what was wrong with me, that was it! She dropped me like a hot potato."

A betrayal of that magnitude hurts. Joan said that she had no idea why her friend deserted her; she never asked. To this day, she doesn't know. "You find out who your friends are when you get leukemia," she said.

Rose went back to boarding school after two abdominal operations. She spent most of her senior year on chemotherapy but missed very little school. "There were some days when I felt too sick to do anything, so I stayed in bed, but most of the time, I made it."

The loneliness was the worst part. Rose is not a person who develops intimate relationships easily. "I'm very private," she said. "I always have been."

She told very few people, either classmates or teachers, that she had cancer. "My roommate knew, of course, and a few close friends, but I didn't go around talking about it to everyone."

Part of Rose's reticence sprang from her already-established personality, but part was a result of not knowing just how very sick she was. "It never occurred to me that I could die from this," she said. "I mean, I knew there was something really wrong because I had had two operations and was taking all these heavy-duty drugs, but I never thought of myself as having a fatal illness."

It wasn't until Rose was 28 years old and had been well for almost a decade that she was struck by the fact that she had had an illness from which many, if not most, people died. "I was glancing through *Newsweek* one day and saw this story about children who had recovered from cancer. It said that most of us used to die, and it was only recently that a significant number survived.

"I was so shocked that I didn't know what to do. That was the very first time that it *really* hit me how sick I had been."

But at the time, while she was in high school and still receiving treatment, and even when she went off to college and felt better but not yet "cured," Rose was lonely because she felt different from her peers. She *was* different. She had cancer and her classmates did not.

Although adolescents need to be treated in a pediatric facility because of the staff's special abilities, most pediatric oncology units have rooms set aside for older patients. It is extremely important for adolescents to take part in discussions and decisions about their treatment. They ought to be shown their X rays and laboratory reports and informed of plans for the future.

To give teenagers some semblance of control over their lives, their school and social schedules need to be taken into account as much as possible when outpatient treatments are planned. Perhaps most important, they need to be kept informed about the treatment: whether it is working and why change might be contemplated.

Teenagers are great risk takers. A normal part of growing up is testing limits and establishing a sense of one's abilities and prowess. It is not uncommon for adolescents to behave erratically during cancer treatment—and to take dangerous and unrealistic chances by missing clinic appointments and "forgetting" to take oral medication. Parents and clinic staff need to be on the lookout for such behavior and, should it appear, to confront adolescents with what they are doing.

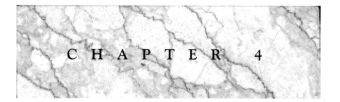

What Cancer Is

One way to control the fear of childhood cancer is by learning about it and understanding how the disease behaves. However, there may be a point at which the books should be set aside because some people grow numbed and frightened by more facts than they can absorb and handle. But others want to know everything that's going on, from basic facts right down to the precise dose of each drug given to their child. There is no "correct" amount of information to acquire, and there is no "right" way of doing things. Some parents and adolescents will spend hours in a medical library poring over texts. Others will feel that the information provided in this book will suffice.

Carcinogenesis

The word *cancer* refers to a process, or a variety of different diseases, rather than to one specific disease. It occurs when a cell, or a group of cells, begins to grow and multiply in a disorganized and uncontrolled way. Each type of cancer primarily affects certain tissues or organs but can spread *(metastasize)* to other tissues and organs.

Carcinogenesis, the cause and origin of cancer, is the major unsolved puzzle in the study of the second leading killer in the Western world (cardiovascular disease is first). Scientists now know that a wide variety of both chemicals and radiation can cause cancer, but they are only beginning to understand the precise causative mechanisms. The ultimate question remains: What is it about radiation, or certain chemicals or microorganisms, such as viruses, that make normal cells turn cancerous?

Radium and X rays were discovered in the 1890s, and right from the beginning of their medical application, people who worked with them noticed dryness, ulcers, and cancers of their hands. But it wasn't until 1910 that a scientist deliberately gave a rat cancer by exposing it to radium. That same year, researchers proved that certain substances (such as viruses) can be a direct cause of certain types of cancer.

Five years later, two Japanese investigators produced skin cancer on the ears of rabbits by repeated applications of coal tar. Since then, dozens of other chemicals have been implicated in the disease.

During the period between the two world wars, and after World War II, research clearly showed that there are pathways of cancer causation—that is, certain chemicals cause cancers of a certain type, and many chemicals produce different types of cancer, depending on the length and type of exposure, the species or strain of animal used in the experiment, and the type of food fed to the animal.

Carcinogenesis implies a relationship between a certain factor (for example, a chemical, a virus, or radiation) and the appearance of cancer. Most early research began as a result of studies that showed that workers who handled certain chemicals had a higher-than-average risk of developing cancer—for example, bladder cancer from dyes and lung cancer from asbestos.

During the 1930s, scientists became interested in the nutritional aspects of carcinogenesis, particularly exposure to hydrocarbons and the metabolism of amino acids. By 1950, interest in nutrition and cancer had all but disappeared. At present, because of new evidence, it is believed that nutrition and cancer are inextricably linked, and the National Cancer Institute is once again investigating the connection between diet and cancer. There is mounting evidence that certain substances in food increase cancer risk. Some nutrients and additives used in food processing (for instance, compounds from nitrites used as preservatives in packaged meat and other foods) may act as contaminants. However, research of this type is still in its earliest stages.

By the end of World War II, even with scientists' ability to cause cancer in laboratory animals, the precise mechanism of carcinogenesis remained a mystery. Puzzling, too, was why some experimental animals exposed to a chemical did not get cancer, and why, for example, some workers in a particular dye factory where everyone was exposed to the same chemical remained cancer free.

At the end of the war, cancer research blossomed. Perhaps because of the bombings of Nagasaki and Hiroshima, and perhaps because of the increasing use of radiation as a medical diagnostic and therapeutic tool, scientists became interested in the carcinogenic properties of ionizing radiation.

Ionizing radiation occurs in two main forms: electromagnetic rays (X rays and gamma rays) and subatomic particles (neutrons, protons, pions, and alpha and beta particles). Natural radiation comes both from outer space (cosmic) and from under the earth's crust, the latter in the form of radium and radon gases resulting from the decay of uranium and thorium. There is nothing anyone can do about natural radiation; it simply exists.

Sources of artificial radiation include television sets, some fertilizers, building materials, and machines used for medical procedures. The last is by far the largest source for most people (discounting nuclear detonations and accidental serious leaks from nuclear power plants).

There is little doubt that exposure to *enough* radiation is carcinogenic. Some tissues are more susceptible than others, but once a cell has been exposed to a high-enough dose of radiation, the process of carcinogenesis is similar to that initiated by exposure to chemicals. One major problem, however, is knowing how much radiation is dangerous.

In 1953, cancer research took a giant leap forward when Watson and Crick discovered the structure of deoxyribonucleic acid (DNA), the molecule that controls the essential life processes of all cells through the genetic information it contains. The arrangement of the molecular compounds on the twisted DNA strand is what determines heredity and cell function, much as a computer program determines what appears on the screen. An alteration in the normal arrangement usually means trouble: either a genetic disorder or a disease such as cancer.

By 1957, scientists were able to induce in laboratory animals almost every form of cancer, many of which were strikingly similar to their human counterparts. However, some animals exposed to a carcinogen developed cancer in sites other than the place of direct exposure. For example, mice exposed to certain hydrocarbons got lung cancer as well as a tumor at the site of the injection. This phenomenon led to research programs investigating the various pathways by which the process of carcinogenesis is activated.

Once scientists knew that all cancers begin in a single cell and that DNA controls the hereditary characteristics of all cells, they could begin to ask questions about the role played by DNA in turning normal cells cancerous. Perhaps, for example, a carcinogen affects DNA in such a way that it gives a faulty or misleading genetic message to all the cells into which the original cell divided. In other words, a carcinogen may cause the DNA to malfunction.

One major difference between a normal cell and a cancerous one is the way it divides. The latter does not stop dividing. Whereas normal cells divide until there is a sufficient number to either repair damaged tissue or replace dead cells, cancer cells lack the mechanism to "know" when that point has been reached, probably because the DNA in these cells has been mutated by a carcinogen. So they reproduce indefinitely.

This discovery led scientists to believe that carcinogenesis is a two-stage process, the first of which is an immediate (sometimes within a few hours) and irreversible change in the cell following exposure to the culprit carcinogen. The second stage results from exposure to other chemicals.

By the mid-1970s, it was possible to identify hundreds of chemical carcinogens and to explain how humans exposed to them developed cancer. It also became evident that subtle differences in chemical compounds determine whether they are carcinogenic. In other words, very small molecular changes in a chemical can mean the difference between carcinogenesis and normal cell functioning.

Further study of DNA led researchers to realize that there is a strong genetic component in carcinogenesis. People differ in their response to carcinogens, and that difference may be familial—that is, some cells may be genetically predisposed to cancer. For example, the genetic disease xeroderma pigmentosum is a rare mutation that prevents DNA from correcting gene damage inflicted by ultraviolet light. Thus, people with xeroderma pigmentosum are especially prone to skin cancer. In fact, they are almost guaranteed to get it on even slight exposure to ultraviolet light.

The immune system also plays a role in carcinogenesis. This complex system is the body's defense against outside invaders such as viruses, bacteria, and other microorganisms. The immune system may also protect us against ourselves—that is, it may prevent normal cells from turning cancerous. Or, as in the case of cancer, it may fail to act.

The role of the immune system in carcinogenesis is only now beginning to be explored, but the discovery of monoclonal antibodies in the mid-1970s opened new avenues of research. An antibody is a protein molecule manufactured as a reaction to *antigens*—foreign protein substances. Production of antibodies is crucial to the function of the immune system. Antibodies are antigen-specific—that is, an antibody binds to only one type of antigen and thus "tags" it for identification and destruction by other cells in the immune system. The "trick" in the production of monoclonal antibodies is to manufacture antibodies that could be made to tag *only* certain antigens—for example, those produced by cancer cells. Study of the way antibodies behave can provide clues about the way cancer cells behave.

Metastasis occurs when a minute piece (sometimes only a few cells) of an original tumor breaks off and is carried by the blood or lymph stream to other areas of the body. These tumor cells attach themselves and establish a "colony" that can eventually exceed the parent tumor in size and ferocity. The most frequent sites for metastasis are the lymph nodes near the original tumor, the lungs, the long bones in the arms and legs, the spine, ribs, liver, skin, and the brain.

Diagnosis

The signs and symptoms of cancer vary so much, and are usually so insidious at first (joint pain or swelling, low-grade fever, fatigue, pallor, or loss of appetite, all of which vary with the type of cancer and how far advanced it is), that the disease may develop for some time before parents realize that something is wrong, and before it is recognized and diagnosed by a physician.

Diagnosis can be simple or it can tax all the skills of physicians who specialize in cancer (oncologists). It all depends on the site and the extent of the disease. The challenge is to detect the cancer as early as possible, when cure is most likely.

Some tests are fairly routine, such as having blood drawn or urinating into a sterile bottle; others, such as a spinal tap or bone marrow biopsy, require special equipment and anesthesia. The word *routine* can be accurately applied either to the hospital personnel's procedures, because they have done the tests so many times before, or to the tests themselves, because they are so common. But when one gives a sample of one's own body cells, or watches while a test is done to one's child because cancer is suspected, the whole procedure jumps out of the realm of routine and into the sphere of the truly terrifying. In fact, some parents and older children say that waiting for the test results is one of the worst parts of the diagnostic process.

The only sure way to establish a cancer diagnosis is by examining the blood, urine, cerebrospinal fluid, lymph, bone marrow, and/or the tumor itself. Each one of the many types of diagnostic tests culminates in actually looking at the child's cells under a microscope. This procedure is called a *biopsy*.

There are three ways to perform a biopsy: excision (removing the entire tumor), incision (cutting into the tumor to remove some of the cells), and aspiration (inserting a needle into the tumor and drawing cells out into a syringe—the "opposite" of giving an injection).

Many parents are familiar with ultrasonography. In fact, they have probably seen a sonogram of their child as a fetus. Ultrasonography is used to locate and "see" a tumor in the same way that it locates and "sees" a fetus.

Ultrasonics are sound waves above the frequency detectable by the human ear, even above those used in dog whistles. By passing these waves through different kinds of materials (such as human tissue), properties such as density, porosity, viscosity, and even chemical composition can be determined. Because tumors often have a density different from that of the normal tissue in which they are located, the reflecting ultrasonic waves will create a "picture" (the sonogram) that delineates the tumor and can even pinpoint its position and dimensions, just as a pregnant woman can watch her fetus move inside her while ultrasonography is being performed.

In addition to the tests that many people are at least somewhat familiar with from watching medical programs on television or reading newspapers and magazines, some diagnostic procedures are more exotic—and expensive.

A CT (computerized tomography) scan—also called a CAT (computerized axial tomography) scan—is a special X-ray technique in which minor differences in the body's absorption of X rays can be enhanced by computer. Instead of standing in front of an X-ray plate (as one does for a chest X ray, for example), the patient is put into a machine that looks much like a gigantic doughnut. The X-ray beam rotates around the patient's body and strikes detectors on the other side of the tube from which the beam originates. These detectors convert the X rays into electrical signals, and a computer analyzes the signals and builds an image that can be viewed on a computer screen or converted into still pictures.

Just as an ordinary X ray doesn't hurt, neither does a CT scan. The machine, however, can be intimidating, even for an adult, so parents should insist that the procedure be thoroughly explained to a child. If possible, the parents and the child should visit the X-ray department so that the child can see the machine before his or her test.

CT scanning is particularly beneficial in examining soft tissue because traditional X-ray machines are not sensitive enough to distinguish among various densities of soft (nonbone) tissue. A CT scan can also detect abnormal tissue inside very dense organs such as the liver.

NMR (nuclear magnetic resonance), also called MRI (magnetic resonance imaging), is a highly sophisticated technique in which the spin of particles (protons) in a magnetic field is measured after a radiofrequency current has been applied. A computer measures the rate at which the spinning particles return to where they were before the current was applied. No X rays are used.

CT and NMR are not painful and they involve no invasive instruments such as needles or scalpels. But they can be frightening for the child (even adults say they experience a great deal of anxiety during these tests) because he or she must be alone in the room where the test is being done, the machinery is huge, and the procedure involves being slid on a stretcher through an opening to the center of the machine. Many people find the experience lonely and claustrophobic, even though they are always in voice contact with the technicians in the control room, who can see everything through a plate glass window.

PET (positron emission tomography) uses a computer to measure the decay of certain isotopes that have been injected into the body. This technique is used to determine the metabolism of the organ being examined, usually the brain, because tumor cells have a different metabolic rate than normal cells. PET can thus help determine how a cancer behaves as well as where it is located.

After a tumor is identified and examined by biopsy, it is "staged"—that is, evaluated for the extent of the disease. Staging is a process for classifying the disease in order to establish treatment guidelines. Three factors are taken into account when cancer is staged: the nature of the primary tumor, the condition of the surrounding lymph nodes, and the extent of the metastasis. Staging is more helpful for certain types of cancer than for others.

Cancers Most Common in Children

Cancer is usually distinguished and named either by the part of the body or organ system it attacks or by the type of cells from which it arises. In addition, the age of the child is often associated with the type of cancer. For instance, retinoblastoma, neuroblastoma, and Wilms' tumor are most likely to occur in very young children—those younger than 3 years of age. Brain tumors and cancers of the central nervous system are seen most often in 5- to 10-year-olds. Bone cancers and lymphatic cancers usually occur in older children and adolescents. Leukemia is first diagnosed most often in children between the ages of 2 and 12.

Leukemia

Leukemia, the most common childhood cancer, is characterized by uncontrolled proliferation of immature lymphoid cells (a type of white blood cell) that originate in the bone marrow. The rapid growth of leukemic cells in the marrow overwhelms healthy blood cells and infiltrates the bloodstream, from whence it can metastasize. There are two major types of leukemia: chronic leukemia and acute lymphoblastic (or lymphocytic) leukemia (ALL). There are also a variety of non-lymphocytic types of leukemia (ANLL). Most leukemias have at least a 75% cure rate if diagnosed early and treated aggressively.

ALL, with about 2,000 new cases a year in the United States, represents one-third of all childhood cancers. Its incidence peaks at 4 years of age. Early symptoms include anorexia (loss of appetite), weight loss, pallor, fatigue, fever, and petechiae (broken capillaries that show as small red spots on the skin).

There is a definite relationship between age at diagnosis and prognosis; treatment of children younger than 2 or older than 10 years of age who are diagnosed with ALL is less effective than treatment of those of ages in between, although the prognosis for all ages of children with ALL is improving every year.

Treatment for ALL usually consists of a combination of chemotherapeutic drugs to reduce the number of leukemic cells. For 95% of patients, the first burst of chemotherapy produces the desired effect. A maintenance regimen of a different combination of drugs is then instituted, and sometimes radiation to the head is given to prevent metastasis to the brain and spinal cord. Although the length of treatment and the types of drugs used vary, most children are in active treatment for about 2 years and on maintenance treatment for another 2.

ANLL has a lower rate of cure (40%) than ALL, but it is also less common—only about 500 new cases a year are diagnosed in this country. The symptoms and treatment are similar, although the combinations of drugs used are different.

Chronic leukemia affects mature cells rather than immature ones, and its onset is slow compared with ALL. It is rare in childhood; in fact, chronic leukemia represents only 5% of all childhood leukemias.

Brain Tumors

Tumors of the central nervous system, usually in the brain, are the second most common childhood cancer, most frequently seen in 5- to 10-year-olds. There are about 1,200 new cases a year in the United States. Brain tumors account for 20% of all pediatric malignancies.

Symptoms depend on the size and location of the tumor, but most arise from two major phenomena: compression and distortion of normal brain structures, and increased intracranial pressure. Both types of symptom occur as a result of the encroachment of the tumor. Common symptoms include morning headache accompanied (and sometimes relieved) by vomiting, personality changes, increasingly poor academic performance, vague headaches throughout the day, and fatigue.

If operable, the tumor is removed surgically and then radiation and sometimes chemotherapy are administered. However, the latter is not especially effective in treating brain tumors because of the existence of the blood-brain barrier. This is a natural phenomenon that prevents substances that circulate in the body's bloodstream from entering the brain's circulation. It is nature's way of protecting the most important and delicate organ from a variety of toxins, but in the case of chemotherapy, the usefulness of the blood-brain barrier "backfires" and prevents drugs from reaching their target.

Computed tomography (CT) scans and magnetic resonance imaging (MRI) have significantly improved the ability to localize tumors, thereby enabling both surgery and follow-up radiation therapy to be much more sophisticated and effective. The location of the tumor and the amount of normal tissue invaded determine the long-term outcome of the treatment and its aftereffects. For example, patients with tumors of the brain stem have a very poor prognosis, and astrocytomas (tumors arising from *astrocytes,* a type of cell found in the brain) tend to grow very quickly and to be resistant to complete surgical removal and curative radiotherapy.

Bone Cancer

Osteogenic sarcoma—cancer of the bone—primarily affects adolescents and young adults, usually during their growth spurt in the second decade of life. It more often affects taller than shorter youths. (It is interesting to note that big dogs, such as Great Danes and St. Bernards, get osteogenic sarcoma 185 times as often as small dogs.)

The prognosis depends both on the extent of the disease at diagnosis and on the type of tumor. The more the cancer has metastasized, the worse the outcome. Prognosis also is affected by the primary site of the tumor: If the cancer arises first in the long bones of the limbs, the outcome is more favorable than if it occurs first in what is known as the axial skeleton (the skull, vertebrae, pelvis, and other flat bones).

Treatment consists of surgical removal of the tumor, which also can mean amputation of the limb, followed by chemotherapy. The extent of the surgery depends on the site of the tumor, the degree of metastasis, the age of the child, and the degree of bone development, as well as on the child's personality factors.

Limb salvage is often possible, and various types of metallic devices and biologic grafts can be used to preserve function. If a limb has to be amputated, the child is fitted with an artificial limb (prosthesis) shortly after surgery. Most children adapt to a prosthesis easily, although the psychological effects of amputation are not as easy to cope with.

Ewing's sarcoma is another type of bone cancer, also seen most often in the second decade of life. Metastasis to the lung is common. Since about half of all children with this form of cancer already have metastasis at the time of diagnosis, chemotherapy prior to surgery is almost mandatory. This accomplishes two things: It shrinks the tumor and gives doctors an opportunity to assess the child's reaction to the drugs.

The goal of treatment is, of course, to preserve as much function as possible so that if the tumor is inaccessible or if the surgery would be too radical (for instance, complete removal of a hip, called a *hemipelvectomy*), intensive radiation therapy—or even total body irradiation—can be substituted. Ewing's sarcoma is considered highly responsive to both radiation and chemotherapy.

Non-Hodgkin's Lymphoma

In contrast with cancer that arises in one specific organ or tissue and metastasizes from there, non-Hodgkin's lymphoma (NHL) is a cancer of the cells that constitute the immune system and that circulate through the entire body. It occurs more often in children who have either a congenital or an acquired deficiency of the immune system. It may be genetic in origin. NHL also might be the result of a viral infection, perhaps by the human T-cell leukemia virus (HTLV), Type I or Type II.

Although the *neoplasm* (literally, "new tissue") affects the immune system in general, a tumor may grow in a specific lymph node. Thus, the symptoms depend on the location of the tumor. For example, if the tumor is in the chest, the child might have chest pain or a swelling under the skin. If the tumor is in the abdomen, he or she will have stomachaches and possibly bowel movement changes.

Treatment consists of chemotherapy. More than two-thirds of all children with NHL survive.

Hodgkin's Disease

Hodgkin's disease—cancer of the lymph system—is the result of the appearance of certain cells (Reed-Sternberg cells) that are not seen in normal tissue. It has about the same survival rate as leukemia. As with non-Hodgkin's lymphoma, this type of cancer is common in people with an underlying immune deficiency. Symptoms include painless enlargement of lymph nodes (most noticeable are the ones under the lower jaw), fatigue, weight loss, and anorexia. Hodgkin's disease is often diagnosed by removal and examination of the spleen and the abdominal lymph glands. It is treated with radiation and combination chemotherapy.

Wilms' Tumor

Wilms' tumor, a cancer of the kidney, is seen most often in 2- and 3-month-olds. There are about 350 new cases diagnosed each year in the United States. Treatment is usually so successful that many children recover completely and have no noticeable effects by the time they are old enough to start school.

The cancer starts before birth (i.e., a *gestational* or *embryonal* tumor) and rarely metastasizes. The diseased kidney is removed and chemotherapy is given, sometimes along with radiation. The child can function well for the rest of his or her life with only one kidney. Once in a while, if the tumor is exceptionally large, chemotherapy and/or radiation is given prior to surgery to reduce its size.

Neuroblastoma

Neuroblastomas, the most common nonbrain tumors of childhood, are sympathetic nerve cell tumors usually located in the chest, neck, or abdomen (the most common origin is the adrenal gland). The sympathetic nervous system controls many involuntary body functions such as digestion and respiration. This type of cancer has a definite genetic component, and it is not unusual to see siblings and identical twins with neuroblastomas. The tumor is removed surgically and followed with radiation and/or chemotherapy, depending on the stage of the disease.

Neuroblastomas most often affect very young children (the average age is 2 years). Survival is much more likely when the disease is diagnosed before 1 year of age.

Rhabdomyosarcoma

Rhabdomyosarcomas are tumors of the muscles, cartilage, and other connective tissue that arise from embryonic tissue, but their cause is unknown. They occur most often in young adolescents and account for 5%–8% of all childhood cancers. The prognosis depends on the extent of the disease at the time of diagnosis.

Because rhabdomyosarcomas metastasize easily, preoperative chemotherapy is given to shrink the tumor before it is removed surgically and before more chemotherapy and/or radiation is administered.

Hepatic and Endocrine Tumors

Liver cancer is extremely rare: it accounts for less than 2% of childhood cancers. Liver and endocrine tumors are gestational or embryonal in nature and thus usually become evident during the first 6 months of life. Endocrine tumors, about half of which arise from the gonads (testicles and ovaries), are usually non-hormone secreting and in many cases develop during the embryonic period.

The tumor must be surgically removed, and, in the case of liver cancer, the entire lobe of the organ is generally taken out with the tumor in order to leave "clean margins"—that is, to remove enough healthy tissue to ensure that all the cancer was removed. However, there are instances in which the tumor is so large that it invades the entire liver. Chemotherapy is given in such cases, and the prognosis is not as good as it would have been had less-radical surgery been successful.

Often, chemotherapy is given preoperatively to shrink the tumor so that more of it (or even the entire malignancy) can be surgically removed.

Retinoblastoma

A retinoblastoma is a malignant tumor of the retina that occurs before birth. Its etiology (cause) is unknown, and although an infant is born with the malignancy, it is not usually diagnosed until symptoms appear. Unfortunately, by the time that happens, the disease is fairly far advanced. The most common symptom is a white spot in the eye.

The disease is rare—only 200 new cases are diagnosed each year—but the treatment is drastic. Although the disease can be cured, it is unlikely that doctors can preserve sight in the affected eye. If the cancer is far advanced, the whole eye must be removed, but if it is caught early, treatment may consist of photocoagulation, cryotherapy, or radiation. If both eyes are affected, surgery is usually not performed.

If the disease has metastasized to the optic nerve, the prognosis worsens, depending on the extent of the spread. If the optic nerve is not involved, the chance of survival is almost 100%.

CHAPTER 5

Treatment

Once the diagnosis has been made, treatment is instituted immediately. The goal of all treatment for childhood cancer is to do as much damage as possible to the cancerous cells while damaging as few normal cells as possible. This chemical balancing act is what causes side effects, because it is impossible for such potent drugs not to have an effect on normal as well as diseased tissue.

Treatment is a time of enormous physical and emotional stress for the child, parents, and siblings. There are always physical discomforts—sometimes only a mild feeling of queasiness, but often severe and debilitating nausea, a wide variety of other toxic side effects, and postoperative pain.

The first phase of treatment involves spending a few days to a few weeks in the hospital having surgery or receiving the initial doses of chemotherapy or radiation. There is usually no need to stay long in the hospital because treatments are done on an outpatient basis, and the child is not sick enough to stay in bed. The child is then discharged, and parents and siblings eventually learn to take care of him or her at home.

Giving medicines is not as fearsome and complex as people believe. Intravenous chemotherapy, of course, is given by doctors and nurses, but oral medicines and injections are easy to learn to give. Hospital home nursing departments and visiting nurse services teach all aspects of home care and act as consultants if there are problems.

Family members also learn to cope with the side effects of the treatment, which become almost routine after a short time. Parents learn how their child reacts to the therapy, how much he or she can eat, and how much sleep is needed. Doctors and nurses know what generally works well when dealing with side effects, but parents learn quickly about their own child's individual needs and desires.

In the end, it is endurance that gets people through. There are ways to increase one's ability to endure and to make the process seem less onerous:

- Use relaxation techniques such as deep breathing and guided imagery to get through complex or painful treatments such as spinal taps or bone marrow biopsies.
- Use hypnosis or behavioral techniques to alleviate some of the side effects of chemotherapy.
- Join patient support groups or talk informally with other patients to learn how other people manage the experience.

Karen went through three bouts of leukemia before she was cured. She was diagnosed when she was 6 years old, and doesn't remember much about the very early times in the hospital. "I think my parents had a lot to do with that. They made jokes and games out of it. I don't remember anything terrible about it, but I suppose everyone has a tendency to block those things out."

Her third bout of leukemia showed up as a mass in her breast. The lump was removed, and she did not need a mastectomy. "I didn't have to be put to sleep for that, so I was able to watch. I find all that stuff very interesting."

Did her intellectual curiosity help her to get through the experience?

"I think my family and friends helped. I really do. They listened to me if I was hurting, but they wouldn't let me dwell on it. There are other things to think about and do. I'm very headstrong, and I think I resented the fact that if I wasn't feeling well one day, I couldn't do what I wanted. I didn't want to be 'that poor little sick kid.' "

She talked about what she remembered of the first hospital experience. "I found a lot of things that went on very interesting, and they weren't necessarily unpleasant. One of the other girls bit a nurse because she didn't want a shot, and that was a big commotion. We used to race up and down the hall in front of the nurses' station, and sometimes we got caught. Some of the children died, but I didn't know it at the time. I was told that they were going away for tests, and then they were put in another room."

Karen described all this in a calm voice, as though she were talking about an ordinary childhood memory. "I had a lot of support. My mother was always there and told me that people were praying for me. When I had to have the fluid removed from my stomach, I screamed during the procedure, but I remember calming down when it was over."

Now in her early 20s, Karen has been cancer-free for 6 years. When asked if she's confident that she's finished with it forever, she said "no" without a moment's hesitation. She believes that the cancer might come back and she has decided to live accordingly.

If the leukemia recurs, Karen will again seek treatment. "If I can beat it three times, I can do it again. I try not to let little things bother me, like when people criticize me. They can be so petty. I try to do everything. I go camping and hiking—everything.

"I think I grew up quicker than other people my age. Different things were important to me. I realized what I'd gone through and how lucky I was. You know, there's more to life than sitting in front of the TV. I just do the things I enjoy and take on new projects all the time."

She'd like to get married and have children. She thinks she can either adopt or perhaps take advantage of new reproductive technology. "You can give birth through your nose these days!" She jokes about it, but beneath the humor lies a belief that if she wants a child, she'll find a way to have one.

Karen doesn't want to miss anything just because she's had cancer.

Surgery

The surgery performed depends entirely on the location of the tumor. That much is obvious. What is less obvious, and what may come as a surprise, is the length of the incision and the number of stitches (or surgical staples) the child will have.

Many types of cancerous tumors are not easily resectable—that is, they cannot be completely removed, either because they are in an awkward location or because they are too large. In these cases, surgery might be postponed while a course of radiation or chemotherapy is given to shrink the tumor and thus increase the likelihood of successful surgery.

Pediatric surgeons are usually willing to describe the nature of the surgery: what will go on inside the body. They are less adept, though, at dealing with the human aspects of the surgery: how bad the pain will be, what the scar will look like, and how long it will take to fade.

Because it is so important for children to be prepared for what will happen to them, parents must insist on getting answers to these questions and whatever others occur to them and their child.

One of the best ways to prepare a child for surgery is to role-play and perform the operation on a doll. The parents, however, must know what is to happen before they can explain it to the child, so they need to be certain that they understand what the surgeon has described. Many pediatric oncology centers have child life therapists who are expert in using toys to teach children and put them at ease.

It is imperative that children be well prepared for surgery. An operating room is probably one of the most frightening places in the world, especially if one is looking at the looming equipment (all of which is spotlessly clean and shiny) and the bustling activity of people who are completely swathed in blue gowns from the tops of their heads to the bottoms of their toes (only their eyes show) from flat on one's back on a stretcher, with a hefty dose of preoperative medication to distort perceptions. The whole experience is incredibly alien, and more than one child has been convinced that he or she has been abducted by space creatures and flown away to another galaxy.

Ben's mother said, "I had my appendix out when I was 15, and I remember how absolutely terrified I was. It wasn't because I was afraid of the machines and the lights and all that—I was old enough to know better, but it was the *atmosphere*. Everyone was busy; everyone looked alike in those funny clothes; no one spoke to me except to ask my name before they wheeled me in; no one smiled. It was incredibly grim. And on top of that, I had this nasty pain in my stomach.

"So I can imagine what poor little Ben went through before his operation, even though we talked about it many times. Poor baby!"

Surgery is a terrible time for parents too. They cannot be with their child during the operation, and there is nothing they can do but sit in the waiting room, drink bad hospital coffee, and worry. There is no way around it. It simply has to be endured.

But when the operation is over, some semblance of control returns. First, they receive information right away. Either the operation went as planned, or it did not. Either way, they know.

Second, they can once again be with their child when he or she returns to the pediatric unit after spending time in the recovery room. Children regain consciousness in the recovery room, and parents cannot be with them there, but they are fully awake when they return to their own rooms, and they should find their parents there to greet them.

Everyone who wakes up from general anesthesia is befuddled, usually in pain from the effects of the surgery, and badly in need of mothering. Grown men have been known to call for their mommies right after an operation, and little children, regardless of their age and developmental level, *need* their mommies and daddies at this time.

Many physicians tend to prescribe too little pain medication for children. It is a widely held myth that children do not feel pain as acutely as adults and that they forget it quickly. Both assumptions are wrong. There is no need to be afraid of providing adequate pain relief after surgery—or for any aspect of childhood cancer. No matter how long the pain lasts, there is no danger of the child's becoming addicted to or tolerant of narcotic analgesic drugs. That is another myth. Unfortunately, there are still doctors and nurses who believe these myths, and it may be up to the parents to insist that their child be given enough pain medication to have a real effect.

Recovery from surgery is usually rapid. Patients are out of bed and walking almost immediately—depending, of course, on the nature of the operation. The more a patient moves around postoperatively, the less the danger of infection and lung problems. Even children with amputations are gotten out of bed very soon. The rehabilitation process begins right away, and as soon as the stump heals, measurements are made for an artificial limb.

Chemotherapy

Chemotherapy often works better in children than adults, especially when drugs are used in combination with one another. These agents' *cytotoxic* effects—that is, the way the drugs kill cancer cells by interfering with the synthesis or function of DNA—are most pronounced in tumors that have a high percentage of actively proliferating cells. These tumors are typical of cancers that affect children.

The response to chemotherapy is sometimes unpredictable. Although it is true that many children respond very favorably very quickly (otherwise, the cure rate would not have improved so dramatically in recent years), it is also true that some children are *resistant* to some drugs—that is, the drugs have less effect than anticipated. Resistance can occur right away or at any time during treatment. Doctors are not certain why this phenomenon takes place, but they believe that it might have a genetic basis. Often the resistance can be overcome by trying other drugs or combinations of drugs. Sometimes nothing works.

Among the many drugs used in the treatment of cancer are vincristine (Oncovin), vinblastine, prednisone, L-asparaginase, methotrexate, 6-mercaptopurine, cyclophosphamide (Cytoxan), Endoxan, daunorubicin, doxorubicin (Adriamycin), procarbazine, bleomycin, Actinomycin-D, nitrogen mustard (Mustine), MOPP (a combination of vincristine, nitrogen mustard, procarbazine, and prednisone), COPP (a combination of vincristine, cyclophosphamide, procarbazine, and prednisone), and MDP (a combination of doxorubicin, vincristine, cyclophosphamide, procarbazine, and prednisone).

Drugs are chosen on the basis of the type of tumor that needs to be treated (its *histology*) and the extent of the disease (the *stage*). General goals of chemotherapy fall into four categories:

& Induction of remission—killing as many cancer cells as soon as possible so that the child enters a disease-free state

- ๑ Central nervous system (CNS) preventive treatment—killing cancer cells that tend to hide in "sanctuary sites" such as the brain and spinal cord
- ๑ Consolidation of treatment—intensifying treatment to reduce the chance of resistance to chemotherapy
- ๑ Maintenance treatment—administering ongoing chemotherapy that lasts for 2 or 3 years after remission is achieved

As soon as the doctors decide on the type of chemotherapy to be used, they insert a permanent indwelling catheter (the two most common are Broviac and Hickman). The plastic tubing is introduced in the chest or abdomen and runs along under the skin until it enters the bloodstream at the jugular or cephalic vein. All medications are given through this catheter (sometimes another tube runs alongside it if one is needed to draw blood samples) so that the child does not need to have a needle stick every time he or she receives a dose of chemotherapy. The place that the catheter enters the skin is kept covered with gauze, and in no time at all the child gets used to the catheter's presence.

Remission

Remission means that the cancer has disappeared for a time, either spontaneously (which happens often enough not to surprise anyone anymore) or as a result of medical treatment.

If the remission lasts 5 years or more without treatment (that is, if there is no evidence of cancer during that time), one is considered to be in permanent remission—cured.

When a child has been in remission for a long time, everyone hopes that this time it's permanent, that this time the cancer is truly gone. Often it *is* gone, but sometimes it is not, and treatment must begin again.

Recurrence means that the cancer has reappeared. If the cancer recurs, patients and their parents go through the entire gamut of emotional reactions all over again. It's usually worse this time, though. Although the element of shock may be blunted, hope is dashed—for a time, anyway.

Side Effects

Anticancer drugs are designed to affect fast-growing tumor cells, but they also have an effect on other fast-growing body tissue such as mucous membranes and hair. This is why so many children suffer from mouth ulcers and why their hair falls out.

The physical side effects of chemotherapy, which also include nausea and vomiting, decreased appetite, and fatigue, are usually only temporarily disabling, although their severity depends on the dose of the drug, the general condition of the child, and often, the attitudes and emotional reactions of the child and parents.

Nausea and vomiting are the most variable side effects. There is no drug that either always or never produces vomiting, and different children react differently to the same drug. In fact, one child will react differently to the same drug at different times. Anti-emetic drugs, given along with or just before the chemotherapy, can prevent the worst of the vomiting, but they also induce severe drowsiness, and some children say they would rather "barf and get it over with than feel zonked out for the rest of the day," as Julia put it.

Some children experience what is called anticipatory vomiting—that is, they throw up either on the way to the hospital or right after arriving there, long before they receive the day's drug treatment. One girl said she vomited every time she drove past the hospital, regardless of whether she was going for treatment. Doctors believe that anticipatory vomiting is a physical rather than a psychological reaction to chemotherapy and is simply a variation of the general reaction to the drugs. Most children who throw up before treatment do not do so again after the drugs are administered.

Some of chemotherapy's most serious side effects are suppression of the immune system and disruption of the number and relationship of various types of blood cells. These render the child vulnerable to infection and hemorrhage.

White blood cells fight infection, and when their numbers drop below a critical level, the child must be isolated from sources of infection, even something as benign as a sneeze or cough. Hospitals are experienced in setting up what is known as "protective isolation," but this environment can be lonely and frightening for both child and parents. For the time during which the child is most at risk, everyone who enters the child's room must wear layers of protective garments over their entire body, including masks over the nose and mouth.

Red blood cells carry oxygen to the tissues, and if their numbers are decreased, the child will be tired and listless.

Platelets are the blood cells that form the body's basic blood-clotting mechanism and react to tissue injuries. If their numbers decrease too much, the child must be protected from injury, which may mean restricting some of his or her physical activities until the platelet count returns to normal.

Sometimes the cancer or the treatment leaves permanent physical marks. Accepting disfigurement is part of survival. For example, Billy can't salivate because of radiation treatments to his neck. So he carries a bottle of water or soda around with him and sips from it occasionally. "Yes, it bothers me, but I don't think about it too much anymore," he said.

Now that thousands of children have survived cancer, many of the long-term effects can be assessed. Chapter 13 discusses some of the enduring physical and emotional consequences of having been treated for cancer in childhood. Again, there is a balancing act to be considered: finding a measure of equilibrium between lifesaving treatment and permanent treatment-induced disabilities.

There are emotional side effects as well. Arthur is 20 years old and has reached the philosophical maturity of an adult—a sensitive, intelligent adult—because he took much of the control of the disease into his own hands. He has thought about some of life's most important and difficult questions and has arrived at answers that most people don't find until their fourth or fifth decade. Did being so sick have anything to do with it?

"Yes, because I've been exposed to reality. Most people who are 19 or 20 don't have to deal with things like that, so I think it's matured me. I feel older than my years. But I think about it only remotely now and don't dwell on it all that much."

When asked if he would go through chemotherapy again, knowing what he knows now about how unpleasant the treatment is, he said he would. "It can be dealt with. I did it before. I could do it again."

Arthur will always be on the way to a goal or in the midst of something important. This time it was school; next time it might be a budding career or a new baby. What if he's "busy" and doesn't want to take time out for months or years of treatment?

"I'll have to wait and see," he replied. "I don't know what my circumstances will be. Maybe treatment will be different then."

Radiation

The goal of radiation is to kill all tumor cells—or at least to decrease the size of the tumor, by interfering with the cells' DNA—without damaging adjacent normal tissue.

Radiation treatment is generally given along with or after a course of chemotherapy to control localized disease. In the past 5 years or so, this treatment has become highly sophisticated. Because tumors can be precisely located by CT scans, the area treated is well defined and there is little damage to normal tissue.

Partial doses of the total radiation dose are administered from several different angles (called *fields*) in order to minimize the damage to normal tissue, through which the rays must pass in order to reach the tumor.

Side Effects

Radiation side effects are either site-specific (reddening of the skin, hair loss, damage to salivary glands, eye irritation) or general (fatigue, bone marrow depression, diarrhea, cystitis).

Children who receive cranial (head) radiation to prevent the spread of leukemia or other cancer to the brain and spinal cord suffer hair loss. Although all children are bothered by baldness to some extent, adolescents, who are very concerned about physical appearance, are the most sensitive about it.

Losing her hair bothered Karen. "It took me a while to get out of the house," she said. But she soon bought a wig and stopped worrying about how she looked. She even got to the point where she could make a joke of it. "When boys would make smart remarks or flirt in an obnoxious way, I just flipped my wig and really shocked them!"

She laughed as she remembered how she coped with her own self-consciousness. She was able to incorporate temporary hairlessness into her life, just as she has incorporated the fact of having leukemia. It had become part of her.

Radiation therapy causes concern about fertility. Karen had been in remission for 13 years when the leukemia showed up again—in her CNS. That news, she said, was "just horrible." She was an adolescent, finished with high school, and just starting out on her own when she had to go through another course of treatment, this time including radiation to her brain and spine.

"I had two choices. One was to start the radiation right away and get a quick start. Another was to move my ovaries aside surgically so the radiation wouldn't affect them. They left that choice to me, and I decided to start right away, so I'm sterile now."

Bone Marrow Transplantation

Bone marrow that is attacked by leukemia and other cancers can be decimated by the disease's damage to cells that divide and replicate quickly, such as blood-forming *stem* (immature) cells. The more virulent the cancer, the more stem cells will die and the more life-threatening will be the consequences.

A bone marrow transplant fills the bones' cavities with healthy marrow from another person to reconstitute the blood-forming and immune systems. As with other human tissue transplants, donor and recipient must be carefully matched. The ideal donor is genetically identical to the recipient—an identical twin. This is called a *syngeneic* marrow graft. Since most people don't have a twin, the next best thing is an *allogeneic* donor—a person whose tissue type is as closely matched to the recipient's as possible.

Tissue typing compares certain genetic characteristics of human leukocyte antigen (HLA), a component of certain body cells. Close tissue-type matches are most often found among close relatives. Nonrelatives can be compatible, but it is difficult to find such individuals and convince them to donate marrow, especially when it is needed quickly.

Children with cancer can be so completely immunosuppressed by massive doses of chemotherapy or radiation that poorly matched transplanted marrow may perceive the recipient's own body tissue as foreign and attack it. This condition—known as graft-versus-host disease—is the most serious complication of bone marrow transplantation. It can be fatal.

Transplants are best done when the cancer is in remission; otherwise, the cancer cells will attack the new marrow, as they did the old, and the transplant will have been for nothing.

About a pint to a pint and a half (500–800 cc) of marrow is removed by needle aspiration from the *iliac crests* (the tops of the flaring hipbone) of an anesthetized donor. The marrow is then passed through a stainless steel mesh to remove blood clots, bone chips, and deposits of fat. Marrow cells are separated from unneeded cells, and the marrow is mixed with heparin, a drug used to prevent clots. Finally, the marrow is given to the recipient intravenously, in the same manner as a blood transfusion.

The marrow "homes in" on marrow cavities, where it establishes itself. In about 2 or 3 weeks, it begins to produce new stem cells, which in turn give rise to red and white blood cells and platelets.

Except for the usual risks that accompany general anesthesia and a remote possibility of infection from the multiple needle sticks to remove the bone marrow, the donor suffers no ill effects. There is no risk of infection as a result of losing marrow cells because not enough are removed to hamper the immune system. Furthermore, since new stem cells form continuously, the donated ones are quickly replaced. About a pint of blood is removed during the process of donation; for this reason, the donor is usually given a pint or two of packed red blood cells (blood cells with the plasma—the liquid in which they are suspended—removed) after the procedure.

Before the bone marrow is transplanted, as many of the recipient's cancer cells as possible must be destroyed. This is done by total body irradiation and high-dose chemotherapy—treatment that puts the patient at high risk of infection because it also suppresses the immune system.

The "trick" is to protect the patient from exposure to infection after the massive cancer treatment until the new marrow begins producing white blood cells. Says Dr. Sanford Leikin, former chief of hematology and oncology at Children's Hospital National Medical Center in Washington, D.C., "A person can live at least 2 or 3 weeks without bone marrow *if* they don't get an infection. It's risky business, but many patients don't have any other hope."

The success rate for bone marrow transplants has improved significantly in the past several years. The chance of success depends on the age of the patient, the type of cancer, and the stage of the disease. Major complications include the following:

- Recurrence of the disease, especially if the transplant was done while the patient was not in remission
- Slow recovery of the immune system, which results in particular susceptibility to viral, bacterial, and fungal infections
- Interstitial pneumonitis (a type of lung inflammation), which is the major cause of death in the first 3 months following transplantation
- Graft-versus-host disease, which affects about 40% of all allogeneic graft recipients

Autologous Transplants

One way to prevent graft-versus-host disease and other complications may be an autologous bone marrow transplant: receiving one's own bone marrow. At first glance, this doesn't make sense. After all, the marrow is diseased. But if the cancer cells can be "washed out" of the marrow, transplanting marrow that is not only genetically identical but is *the same as* the patient's is medically logical and works well in many cases.

Autologous transplant has been used successfully for hard-to-treat leukemias and also has potential in the treatment of solid tumors, lymphomas, melanomas, CNS tumors, and soft-tissue sarcomas. It can be especially useful for those for whom a compatible donor cannot be found.

In this procedure, the patient's bone marrow is removed during remission—when there are the fewest cancer cells in the marrow and when tumor cells are the most sensitive to chemotherapy. The marrow is then treated with high doses of chemotherapy and frozen in liquid nitrogen while the patient is given massive chemotherapy and/or radiation. The marrow is thawed, mixed with heparin, and then injected back into the patient. It travels to marrow cavities and sets up normal functioning within 2 or 3 weeks.

Fetal Liver Tissue Transplants

Sometimes it is impossible to find a compatible donor for bone marrow transplantation and the child is not a candidate for autologous transplant. A new technique, which is still experimental and somewhat controversial, has been used with limited success.

During the early part of pregnancy, the fetus's liver is the major source of blood cell production. Only later in gestation is that function gradually transferred to the bone marrow. Thus, when fetal liver tissue is transplanted as if it were healthy adult bone marrow, it begins to function as such and stimulates the recipient's own marrow to produce stem cells.

Moreover, because fetal liver tissue has fewer mature *T-lymphocytes* (a type of white blood cell) than adult bone marrow, there is less likelihood of graft-versus-host disease. Even though only a very small amount of fetal liver tissue is available and the success rate so far has not been overwhelming, continued study seems worthwhile, especially for those (mostly very young) children whose immune systems have totally failed.

Stopping Treatment

The end of treatment is very scary—almost as scary as starting. The patient is cut off from the chemical supports that he or she had come to depend on, and now there's no protection from the cancer.

Amy put it this way: "When Ben went into remission, we were delighted, relieved—almost delirious. Then, when the doctor said that the course of chemotherapy was over, I felt like a 2-year-old who's had her teddy bear ripped out of her arms.

"Of course, I *knew* that treatment would stop at some point. By the time the doctor made the announcement, I was a walking medical encyclopedia. I knew it, but I wasn't *prepared* for the sense of danger that came over me. I felt as if Ben were completely exposed to giant killer elements floating around 'out there,' like we had sent him to the North Pole stark naked. I was terrified."

Ben has been free of cancer for almost 7 years now, but Amy still remembers the feeling of vulnerability. "It's so hard to describe," she said and then compared it to her own experience with a broken ankle. "You spend all those weeks in a cast with your skin itching like crazy, getting more and more cranky. You count the days until the cast comes off, and then when it does, the first reaction is this terrible insecurity.

"My leg felt so *naked* and exposed. Every time I put it down on the floor, it felt like it wobbled all over the place, and I had to stop myself from asking the doctor to put the cast back on. I felt like I wasn't ready to walk without that support.

"So if I felt that way over a broken bone, you can imagine how bad it was when it was cancer—in my *child*."

Arthur made a surprising decision when he began to think about how the treatment was affecting his life. After about a year and a half of chemotherapy, "I found that I wasn't able to lead the kind of life that I wanted to. I had to come here [to Children's Hospital] every 3 weeks, and often I had to stay for a few days. The medicine made me sick.

"I stuck it out for a while and then I thought, I don't want to do this any more. If I die, then I'd rather die living comfortably. So I quit the medicine against the doctors' advice. Luckily, I've been okay so far."

Arthur knew that there was a 5%–10% chance of a relapse, of contracting a different type of cancer, or of developing a late and currently unknown side effect of the chemotherapy. He had doubts about leaving treatment early and made the decision against his family's advice as well as the doctors', but he said he couldn't do everything he wanted to do if he was periodically incapacitated by the effects of the drugs. During his senior year in high school, Arthur was on the tennis team, worked on the newspaper and yearbook, took two courses at a local junior college, and made the National Honor Society. "All this time I was taking the medicine, but I didn't think I could keep up that pace in college—and still be on chemotherapy."

He doesn't regret the decision and justifies having made it: "Even if I do relapse, it will have been worth it because I will have had this time of normalcy to do what I wanted. And I could have gone through the entire 4 years of treatment and *still* relapsed. Taking a chance was—has been—worth it."

Most children do not do what Arthur did. Most wait until they are discharged from treatment by their physicians. And contrary to what they had anticipated, going off treatment may not be the liberation they had hoped.

Beth described her experience by using an analogy similar to the one used by Ben's mother. She broke her leg the year before she came down with acute lymphoblastic leukemia (ALL). She, too, felt insecure when the cast came off.

"Then when the doctor put that plastic air cast thing on, I was glad, although I wouldn't admit it to anyone. It made me feel secure—like I wouldn't fall over when I tried to walk. I limped for a long time afterwards.

"So when I went off chemo, it was like that. I felt as though the drugs were a 'crutch' and that without them, I would get sick again. It was sort of as if I'd never be able to make it on my own."

Stopping treatment is stressful and scary in the same way that finishing psychotherapy or leaving home to go to boarding school or college is stressful and scary. The familiar is comfortable and safe even though it may be difficult and unpleasant.

Alternative Treatment

Alternative treatment for childhood cancer—or for any disease, for that matter—consists of a variety of remedies that fall outside the mainstream of treatment that has been subjected to the usual types of scientific investigation. Most types of alternative medicine have several characteristics in common:

- They are provided by a variety of people, some of whom are licensed physicians, some of whom are out-and-out quacks, and most of whom fall somewhere in between.
- Claimed treatments or "cures" are not subject to scientific quality control or oversight, and have not undergone scientific testing for safety and efficacy.
- Treatment results have not been published in any recognized medical journal, nor do they appear in published texts.
- Many practitioners of alternative medicine say that mainstream practitioners are jealous of them because they have found the cure for a certain disease. Many of these same people accuse the medical press of "suppressing" information about the cure out of a desire to keep their own patients to themselves.
- Most of the claimed treatments or cures consist of naturally occurring substances: dietary regimens, herbs, vitamins, retinoic acid, Laetrile (made of apricot pits), and the like. Although they are not necessarily harmful, neither are they necessarily effective.
- Other common alternative treatments include the use of "devices" that have no known curative medical effects—for instance, "electrical stimulators," strong lights, ultraviolet light, and ultrasound.
- Many practitioners of alternative medicine claim that their treatment will lead to a "miraculous" cure, and most do not acknowledge the possibility of a spontaneous remission and the role of chance.

All of this having been said, the reader should not assume that alternative medicine is, in and of itself, necessarily *bad*. In fact, most of it is physically harmless. The harm occurs when the child is taken out of mainstream treatment (or never started in the first place) and placed under the care of an alternative practitioner who promises the world but delivers nothing.

It is said that faith can move mountains, and perhaps it can. Perhaps faith can cure cancer. But it is by no means a sure thing.

Even the most cynical and traditional practitioner of strictly science-based medicine has witnessed instances of spontaneous remission, either in the aftermath of failed treatment or when there has been no treatment at all. No one knows how or why these remissions occur, but they do. The problem is that their occurrence is entirely unpredictable, even capricious. It may be that God or some higher power has made a decision about whom to heal, but if that is so, then it is best not to interfere with the process—not to second-guess God, so to speak.

There is no religion on earth that claims to understand the will or way of God. No faith healer has figured it out, nor has any television evangelist, priest, minister, or rabbi.

Faith in God's power to heal is an absolutely personal matter. Hope is, too. Both are to be encouraged, but *not* at the expense of doing everything *humanly* possible to cure the child.

Alternative medical practitioners are not known for their proclivity for telling the truth or for providing useful information to parents. In fact, one of their major stocks in trade is to raise hope and then lie about why a cure did not come about as promised. Many of these lies blame the victims.

If and when parents finally realize that an alternative treatment is not working, they give up and seek traditional medicine. By that time, of course, the cancer has progressed and perhaps metastasized, so that the child's prognosis is far worse than it would have been if the parents had sought appropriate treatment from the start. They may have inadvertently contributed to or hastened the death of their child.

Parents who are determined to seek alternative treatment usually will not be satisfied until they have tried it and found that it doesn't work. The urge to do every single thing in the world to help a sick child is understandable and not, in itself, bad. The act is wrong, though, when the child is denied a chance at established treatment.

If parents insist on going outside the mainstream for medical treatment, they should do at least the following:

- Ask the child if he or she wants to do this. Even young children—9 or 10 years old—are quite capable of participating in these kinds of decisions.

❧ Get the alternative treatment in addition to—not in place of—mainstream treatment. If you want to try everything, then do not forgo the treatment that has provided a cure for so many.

❧ Beware of making a major financial commitment that no insurance policy will cover. *Never* pay for treatment in advance, and be very suspicious of a physician or other practitioner who asks you to pay him or her directly for ancillary care, such as room and board at a clinic, transportation, and the like. Find out who owns the treatment facility. If, as is usual, it is the practitioner him- or herself, beware.

❧ Do not consent to treatment from a practitioner who insists that he or she alone be the sole provider of medical care for your child.

❧ Tell your child's doctors what you are doing. They need to know in order to be aware of the effects of the alternative treatments on the ones they are providing. Drug interactions are a serious matter.

CHAPTER 6

Information and Practical Help

One of the best ways to establish control over any situation is to learn as much as one can about it. The expression "knowledge is power" has great relevance for childhood cancer.

Finding out that one's child has cancer will automatically trigger fears and fantasies of the blackest kind, but information about the disease and its treatment can eventually shade those fears into a manageable pale gray. The more one knows about a problem, the better one is able to cope with it. For this reason, becoming actively involved in the treatment and care of one's child reduces the amount of stress and anxiety by focusing free-floating and nameless fears onto practical tasks. The more actively parents are involved in caring for their child, the less time they have to worry about the ultimate effects of the illness.

But where does one turn for medical help? The "easy" answer is "to the best specialist one can find." To a major university medical center that has a large pediatric oncology division. To the most sophisticated physicians who are aware of the latest treatments and who have the most advanced equipment at their disposal.

The problem with the easy answer is that it's not easy at all—nor is it possible for those who are not familiar with the way the health care system works. Most people are not. Neither is it possible for the many millions of people in this country who, for one or a combination of reasons, do not have access to sophisticated health care—or to any care at all.

It is true that new drugs and new combinations of existing drugs, supplemented perhaps with surgery and radiation therapy, are the most effective weapons against childhood cancer. Unfortunately, such innovative treatments are usually available only at major cancer centers and are less likely to be on hand at smaller community hospitals or rural hospitals. To make matters worse, most of these specialized cancer centers are located in metropolitan areas that may be miles from home.

In general, children with cancer do better when they are treated in specialized centers than at community hospitals, especially when a treatment modality is new. Specialty centers have access to the latest research results; they have established treatment protocols based on years of experience with hundreds of patients; they know how to set up systematic methods of inquiry for current and future treatments; and they have a pediatric intensive care unit, access to a blood bank, facilities for protective isolation, radiation oncologists and pediatric surgeons who understand the treatment of children, and advanced laboratories.

Moreover, such centers have ancillary staff who do nothing but work with children with cancer and their families. These nurses, social workers, psychologists, play therapists, and teachers have had years of experience in guiding families through the confusing, and often aggravating, world of medicine, insurance claim forms, sources of financial aid, and the like.

Frequently, the problem lies in getting to such centers in the first place. When a diagnosis of childhood cancer is made by a family pediatrician, he or she may not be aware of the vast network of facilities available for treatment. If the physician has a crowded, busy practice, he or she may not be willing to take the time to refer the child to anyone but a local oncologist who may have no pediatric experience. In some rural communities, there *is* no oncologist—pediatric or otherwise.

Many parents have reported that one of the greatest stressors is dealing with the *fact* of the illness: dredging up the energy to go through the diagnostic process, which is far more complicated than a simple blood test followed by an announcement of bad news. There may be travel to specialized laboratories and overnight stays at the hospital for complex diagnostic tests, not to mention the challenges of learning the ins and outs of how a hospital functions and how to "work" the system.

However, gathering information and learning as much as possible makes it easier to interpret medical information. These activities can also help parents manage the practical problems. For example, a child on chemotherapy will have a number of side effects that can be dealt with at home with relatively simple remedies. But if parents do not know about what to expect, they will panic and want to rush off to the doctor when mouth sores appear or the child's skin turns red. When the parents' fear level goes up, so does the child's. And then everything seems worse.

Some parents have difficulty convincing themselves of the seriousness of their child's illness. Even worse, many have reported that their pediatrician has refused to take seriously symptoms that could be attributable to a vast array of illnesses—from a bad case of the flu to leukemia. Strange muscle lumps are chalked off as the ordinary bumps and bruises of childish roughhousing and joint pain is pooh-poohed as "growing pains."

Friends and relatives mean well when they say, "I'm sure it's nothing," when a mother expresses worry about a symptom that won't go away. A spouse will say, "Is he sick *again?*"—not meaning to denigrate the presence of ill health, but thinking of the doctor's bill to follow. So a trip to the physician is postponed.

Eventually, though, the gravity of the situation must be faced, and a stubborn and ignorant pediatrician is forced to admit that his or her expertise does not cover treating childhood cancer. If the family is lucky, the doctor will make referrals to appropriate specialists. If they are not, they are on their own, perhaps miles from a big city, perhaps unsophisticated in the ways of using friends and family to obtain medical references.

Where does one find a pediatric oncologist? Although perhaps one could find an adequate source of help in the Yellow Pages, this is not the best place to start. Appendix A lists sources of information on childhood cancer.

Relationships With Health Care Providers

Once the child is receiving appropriate care, a new and somewhat peculiar relationship develops: that between the parents/child and the health care system—an alliance of intimacy with total strangers. At least, they are strangers at first.

Although most people find this alliance an uncomfortable, even frightening, experience, a good relationship with those who provide care to the sick child is crucial. Developing a collaborative effort that will ultimately result in the best interest of the child requires work on everyone's part.

The most positive and encouraging aspect of this relationship is that everyone has the same goal: curing the cancer. And although conflicts do occur, most of the time parents and care providers work well together and form a bond of caring that often lasts long after the child's illness is over.

In pediatric oncology centers, conferences are held from time to time between parents and physicians, nurses, social workers, and others who care for the child. (In smaller or less specialized hospitals, these "conferences" are usually convened informally.) Physicians prefer that both parents attend these meetings because they feel that the discussion will be more complete, and more of what is discussed will be retained. In addition, although everyone receives and interprets information differently, at least the care providers can be sure that each parent has been given the same information.

The only problem with this scenario is that it is frequently impossible. The conferences are usually held during the day, when the breadwinner has other responsibilities. It is sometimes the case that this individual's (usually the father's) absence is interpreted as lack of interest—an assumption that is almost always wrong.

Everyone needs to be aware of several components of the relationship between parents and the people who care for the child:

ॐ Conflicts, even out-and-out power struggles, can arise over who knows the child better and who has ultimate control over his or her welfare.

~ The transmission of information—who provides it, how much is revealed, and the amount of time spent talking with parents and the sick child—is extremely important at every stage of treatment.

~ Honesty and clarity of communication work both ways. Parents and care providers each need to feel that the other party is being open and forthright, and that serious issues are not being avoided.

~ Parents generally make an effort to please their child's physicians because they imbue the medical profession with powers that may at times be unrealistic. Physicians come to know this very early in their training and have been accused (often justifiably) of taking advantage of patients' and families' need to please them. This phenomenon should be guarded against because of the long-term nature of the illness, and because of the collegial relationship of all the treatment providers—including parents.

~ It is natural to be intimidated by the amount of new information that one must assimilate quickly—often during a state of severe shock and stress. It is equally natural not to understand everything that one is told the first time around, or even the second or third. Parents should ask to have things explained again and again if necessary, until they are certain they understand. Most nurses and doctors are very patient, but some are not, and it is therefore up to parents to keep asking questions until they are satisfied. Although this may not seem fair (it is, after all, the parents who are paying for the services of the doctors and nurses), it is the reality, and the people who "pester" the most are the people who understand the most about what is happening to their children.

~ Hospitals are businesses and bureaucracies, and some employees may demonstrate a lack of care and sensitivity toward patients and their families. But for the most part, doctors, nurses, social workers, and others who treat children with cancer care about these patients and their families. Parents would do well to think of themselves as having relationships with people, not with the hospital, and they should insist on being treated honestly, politely, and with sensitivity.

~ Parents can and should insist that their child be treated with kindness, warmth, and gentleness. Physical and emotional pain must be acknowledged and dealt with. If medical care is to be discussed in front of the child (preferably *with* the child), both physicians and parents need to be aware of the child's level of understanding and his or her potential for misunderstanding. No treatment plan or medical procedure should be undertaken until the child understands exactly what is going to happen.

ɛ̀ Nurses and parents need to be very frank with one another regarding how much care the parents are willing and able to provide. Mothers and fathers should be assertive enough to maintain their role as parents, but nurses also have to evaluate the parents' competence to care for the child, both in the hospital and later at home.

Nurses and other caregivers have had vast experience with childhood cancer, whereas the ordeal is brand new for the parents, and probably nothing in their lives has prepared them for it. Nurses do not work in pediatric oncology unless they love children and enjoy being around them; therefore, parents can assume that their children will be treated with love and tenderness. But by the same token, the nurses need to feel that parents have confidence in their competence. "I know they're worried sick about their children," said one staff nurse at Johns Hopkins Hospital. "I know they're frightened to death, and I know they're not themselves. But I wish they'd give me credit for knowing what I'm doing—and for *caring* about their kids."

This nurse expressed a wish that parents would have more consideration for the limits placed on her time and energy, and what is in her and her colleagues' power to do. "We're not God," she said. "We can't take away the big bad cancer, but we *can* relieve some of the pain and suffering. I wish they'd just let us do our jobs."

Patients sometimes have different views of what is happening. June said, "I didn't feel as though they treated me like a person. I was just a 'thing' in the bed that they had to do stuff to—stick needles in, get pills down, take to other parts of the hospital. A lot of the time I was really lonesome, but none of the nurses ever came and just talked to me."

June subsequently became a nurse, and she said that she is very conscious of her patients' feelings. "I always call them by their name, and no matter how busy I am, I always try to look at them to see how they're feeling. I try to be sensitive and caring."

She said the bone marrow biopsy was probably the worst thing that ever happened to her. "I still have nightmares about it." The biopsy, actually two of them because the first one was not successful, occurred 22 years ago, and June still shudders and closes her eyes when she talks about it.

"All I can remember is dozens of hands pressing me down. I was yelling and screaming, and the doctor couldn't get the needle into the right place. I kept feeling all these horrible pains shoot down my leg, and the people were mad at me because I was so terrified, and I was mad at them, and that made me scream louder. It was just horrible." She shivered at the memory.

The next day when they tried again, it wasn't so bad. "They got the chief of the service to do it, and they must have given me a tranquilizer or sedative because there weren't so many hands, and I don't remember being as scared. I think it all went pretty quickly."

June has never had to have another bone marrow biopsy. "But if I do, they're gonna have to knock me out cold to do it!" she said. She means it.

When parents need information or are confused about something, they should be assertive without being aggressive or abrasive. When providing physical care to their own children, they should be helpful without intruding into what is properly a nursing role and without insinuating that they could do a better job than the nurses.

Parents should also

- Learn as much as they can about the diagnosis and treatment in order to know what questions to ask
- Ask that things be explained in "regular" language, not "medicalese"
- Keep track of the child's medications and treatments
- Stay with their child as much as possible (almost all pediatric units make provisions for parents to stay overnight in a comfortable lounge chair)
- Help the child develop his or her own relationship with the health professionals
- Understand their own negative and frightening feelings and learn to direct them appropriately

 Create a special relationship with a few staff members on each shift and ask them for help and comfort when needed

 Talk to and make friends with other parents

Children and adolescents have strong feelings about the people who care for them. In general, they want what all of us want in a satisfying human relationship: honesty, respect, and affection.

Most older children say they want to be included in the discussions about treatment, and they surely want to have a voice in what is done to them. Karen said, "I hated it when the doctors talked about me as if I weren't there—when they were right in front of me. It made me feel like I was just a piece of machinery they were fixing."

Children understand more about their caregivers than they are given credit for. Said Bill: "I know they're busy, and I understand that I'm not the only patient on the ward, but what would it cost them to at least look at me and smile and put a little warmth in their voices?"

He was quick to say that not all his doctors were "cold fish." Usually, the older ones who had been working with childhood cancer for a number of years were able to exhibit emotion and to talk to him as if he were a fully developed person—which he was. But some younger doctors and medical students seemed so distant, "as if they didn't want to get involved with me," said Bill. He was probably correct in his assessment when he said that they were "scared of their own feelings about cancer."

Nonprofessional and Informal Help

Families of children with cancer also need to ask for nonprofessional help. Sometimes it's "only" a cup of coffee with a neighbor or friend to sit and talk. Other times it's as much as friends' taking care of the other children for a week while the parents travel to a distant city to be with their sick child in the hospital.

The problem, of course, is that in order to receive help, one has to tell people about the cancer. This is *not* the same as telling people that your child has broken his leg, or even that he was in a terrible automobile accident. There is still a stigma attached to cancer, and although it has taken "second place" in horror to people's reactions to AIDS, it is never easy to predict how people will react to the news of cancer in a family. The uncertainty is magnified when the patient is a child.

Although it is true that some people are still unenlightened enough to believe that cancer is contagious or that it is somehow a "social" disease, most people do not recoil out of a sense of rudeness or a desire to shun. They are simply ignorant and afraid of their own feelings.

"Also, they just don't know what to do," said Brian's mother. "They are so appalled that something like this could happen that they're almost paralyzed." She compared it to a death in the family: "You know how people react when you tell them that your mother died. They can't look you in the eye, they can't seem to say the simplest thing about how sorry they are, and God knows, the art of writing a letter of sympathy seems to be lost forever.

"And that's a short-term thing! When they hear that your child has bone cancer and has to have his leg amputated, they just can't deal with it. So they ignore it, you get all hurt and resentful, and before you know it, the friendship is down the tubes."

This need not happen, but preventing it takes work on everyone's part—and energy that parents may not have. As Brian's mother observed, the experience of childhood cancer can change the very nature of social relationships and even close friendships. "You sure find out who your friends are" is an oft-repeated statement.

It is important to learn how to ask for help and to realize that most people enjoy doing things for others. Amy found this difficult at first. "When I was growing up, my parents always taught me never to ask for favors because it wasn't a good idea to be beholden to people. Then you would be in their debt and that would put you at a disadvantage.

"So I never asked for anything. When I was in my 20s, I was giving a birthday party for a friend, and 2 days before, I slipped on a wet floor in the supermarket and broke my ankle. I went on with the party and never called any of the guests to ask them to come over and do the preparation.

"That attitude is silly, I realize, but it's the way I was. When Ben got sick, I had a hard time talking about my feelings with close friends because I didn't want to burden them.

"My husband traveled a lot on business, and he took so much time off work at the beginning of Ben's illness—he fell apart and was no help to me at all—that later on, he had to make up for all the time lost, so everything fell on my shoulders. The only reason I didn't fall apart was because Ben needed me.

"One day when I was carrying Ben to the car for his chemotherapy, I saw my neighbor cutting his lawn, and without even thinking about it—if I had thought about it, I never would have gotten up the nerve—I went over and asked him to cut my grass. Not only did he do it, but when I got back from the hospital, he had trimmed the shrubs and pulled out the biggest of the dandelions.

"When I went over to thank him, he looked genuinely happy to have been of help, and I believed him when he said to ask for anything I needed."

It took Amy a long time to realize that not only could she ask for help, she liked giving people the opportunity to help her.

Establishing the boundaries of privacy is a crucial task, and you are the only one who can do it. It is impossible for your friends to know how much you want or need to talk about the experience unless you tell them. They may not be able to meet your needs, but they surely cannot if they do not know what those needs are.

If you need help, you must ask for it, either directly or in response to an offer. Many parents are frustrated by "general" offers of help ("If there's anything I can do, please don't hesitate to call") and are unsure of the offerer's sincerity. There is one way to find out and that is to put the offer to a test. Calling someone and saying, "Would you be willing to babysit Friday night for a few hours while Jim and I go out to a movie?" will elicit a definite response.

If your friend agrees immediately—and with grace—you'll know you indeed have a friend. If the refusal is genuine and a counteroffer is made ("I've already made plans for Friday night; how about doing it on Saturday when my calendar is free?"), you likewise have a friend.

Other responses may not necessarily be a complete rejection, and you might want to try again another time. But you will be able to tell from the person's attitude and tone of voice whether the offer was real.

Be specific about what you need. If you were going to ask a friend for a loan, you wouldn't say, "I need some money"; rather, you would request a certain amount of money for a certain period of time: "Could you lend me $50 until the bank replaces my automatic teller card?" The same holds true for other favors:

- Collecting the newspapers and mail while the family is away at the treatment center, *not* "Could you sort of look after things for a while?"
- Picking up your 2-year-old at day care every Monday, Wednesday, and Friday for the month of April while you take your sick child for outpatient chemotherapy, *not* "Would you help take care of Jamie until Brian is finished with chemo?"
- Requesting that a neighbor let you know when she is going to the supermarket and asking her to buy your groceries, *not* "It's such a drag, taking Sam to the store when he's so weak and sick."

Sometimes parents do not even have to ask for help. Leslie Nelson tells the story of a family in Milwaukee and their neighbors: "One day, early in the child's illness, the mother came home from the hospital where her child was undergoing treatment. There, taped to the back door, was a 'sign-up sheet.' It was a big piece of paper divided into a grid by days of the week and by household chores. Neighbors, some of whom the family didn't even know, had signed up to provide dinner once a week, or take the family's garbage to the dump, or cut the grass and water the lawn. Some volunteered to do the weekly grocery shopping and one drove the youngest sibling to and from day care every day."

All it took was one person to think of the idea and coordinate the plan. The rest fell into place as a result of people's natural desire to help others in times of crisis.

One problem, though, with the well-meaning assistance of friends and neighbors, said Nelson, is that "the novelty of the illness wears off after a while. People grow bored with sickness and don't have the emotional stamina to continue their support for the length of the illness."

Parents have expressed similar concerns. Ben's mother said, "During the first month or so, it was great. People sent cards and wanted to visit him in the hospital. Of course, that was when he was the sickest and had a hard time enjoying visitors.

"But as the months passed, Ben being sick got to be 'old hat,' and just as he was starting to feel better, people sort of forgot about him. Oh, I guess they didn't really *forget*, but it was like they were impatient and wanted him to hurry up and get better as fast as someone gets better from measles or a broken bone or something. And when he didn't be-cause he *couldn't*, he was hurt by what he saw as their abandonment. It was hard for me to explain that people still liked him, but that they just didn't understand what he was going through. But he was still hurt—and I don't blame him. I was, too."

Informal groups of parents often form spontaneously in hospital and outpatient clinic waiting rooms. These groups of people, who soon get to know each other intimately, provide emotional support and establish networks of new friends and relationships with people who have similar experiences. Many parents have said that they received more reassur-ance, empathy, and practical help from other parents in the waiting room than they did in formal support groups or even in professional therapy.

"One day in the clinic waiting room, I couldn't hold the tears in one more minute," said Sarah. "I knew, though, that I could cry my eyes out and no one would ask me to explain why. No one told me that things weren't as bad as they seemed, or that everything would be all right. Every single parent in that room knew exactly why I was crying, and I didn't need to feel ashamed or embarrassed."

Other people say that they are grateful to have the opportunity to help others. Brian's mother said, "During his last week of chemotherapy, I met this woman whose baby had just been diagnosed. She was so young, no more than 19 or 20, and so lost in the big medical center. She had come from somewhere way out in the country and hardly knew how to negotiate the parking garage.

"Another mother and I took her in hand and showed her the ropes. We made lists of things she had to do, and wrote down the phone extensions of everyone who could get things done in the pediatric on-cology department. She was staying at the Ronald McDonald House and didn't have a car, so we took her on a tour of the neighborhood so she could learn what was within walking distance. I never saw her again after that first week, but I felt wonderful to have been able to make her life a little easier."

Some people say that as treatment progresses, they are happy to be able to talk to others about how the fact of childhood cancer has changed their lives. "Lots of people tell stories about the positive effect that the cancer had on them," said Brian's mother. "When we first started coming to the clinic, I could hardly believe that people were talking like that, but I decided to listen, and before I knew it, I was telling everyone about how mature Brian had become since he got sick.

"He used to be kind of wimpy at times. . . . Okay, he was a big cry-baby! But now, somehow he's pulled himself together, and if he survives the cancer, I know I won't have to worry about the kind of person he becomes. He'll be terrific because all of a sudden, he *is* terrific."

CHAPTER 7

Help for Parents
and Children

Children with cancer and their parents sometimes feel overwhelmed, drowning in sorrow, rage, and despair. Emotional paralysis becomes more than a way of describing feelings; it turns into reality, forcing lives to a virtual halt. At those times, even one's closest friends and family cannot provide the comfort to get through the darkness.

One mother said she felt so utterly alone and isolated that even her sister, with whom she had shared the greatest intimacy over the years, couldn't help. If she hadn't found a psychiatrist she trusted, she thinks she might have killed herself. "The walls were closing in on me," she said. "I don't know what I would have done if I hadn't had my doctor to call the night I really thought I might get in the car and well, you know . . ."

Another mother said, "You're allowed to talk about the grief and fear for a while but not for as long as you *need* to. I'm not sure at what point people's patience with your troubles begins to wear thin, but it does, and they make it really obvious that they think you ought to snap out of it and get on with things. The only trouble is that I wasn't ready when everyone thought I should be."

Using a combination of internal and external coping strategies—and people do this without being aware of what they are doing—usually works in most situations, and relatively balanced adults have vast experience dealing with the stress and small crises of everyday life by marshalling the coping skills they have developed over the years.

For example, when a child falls off her skateboard and breaks her arm, a parent will adapt internally to the crisis by accepting the fact that the child will be incapacitated and in a sulky mood for a while. There is also optimism that when the cast comes off and the muscles regain their strength, things will return to normal.

The parent's external strategies include solving the problem by taking the child to the emergency room, finding out if specialized treatment is needed, and asking how to care for the broken arm.

When the crisis is cancer, parents immediately fall into their usual patterns of coping, which in this case may not be sufficient. No amount of broken bones and high fevers of common childhood ailments can prepare parents for the mind-numbing terror of what has happened and what lies ahead.

Coping strategies fail or break down in the face of overwhelming crisis, and maintaining emotional balance can become an impossible task. The things that usually work to prevent extreme mood swings from interfering with meeting family obligations and caring for the sick child seem to fly out the window, and the vow to take each day as it comes is broken—which, of course, makes people feel guilty and further interferes with their ability to cope. This may be the time to realize that the strength of one's feelings, while entirely natural, has gotten out of control. It is time to get professional help.

Since the agony of grief and pain is universal, seeking professional help is not a shame or a failure of character. In fact, it shows the opposite. Making that phone call for help is a strong, positive statement about determination and will.

Koocher and O'Malley (1981), in their interviews with parents of children who survived cancer, asked parents what kind of help they would have found beneficial while their child was ill. Most said they would have liked to have been referred to a mental health worker as a routine part of the treatment plan. They did not feel as though they had been rendered mentally ill or incompetent by the presence of the illness, but it would have been advantageous to have been able to talk to someone who could tell them how other people reacted and coped in similar circumstances.

Specifically, the parents wanted to see someone during the first week or so of the illness and they wanted to know what the common issues were so that they would have some idea of what to expect. Even people who did not, as a rule, talk about their feelings said they would have made an exception in this case.

The lesson to be learned, then, from what these parents said is that if emotional help is not offered by the pediatric oncology team (in most large medical centers it is), parents need to ask for it.

As in finding help of all kinds, it is best to ask others for referrals. The hospital's social service department is a good place to start. But if there is no one there that you wish to take into your confidence, tell a close friend or two, perhaps someone who you know has been in therapy, that you need counsel.

Counseling Professionals

Clergy

Some priests, ministers, and rabbis provide therapy if they have been trained in pastoral counseling. If not, a clergyperson is a good source of referral. You are not the first member of the congregation to ask for help, nor will you be the last. Almost all congregations of any size have referral lists of community resources of all types, including mental health professionals.

Many people ask God for help. Some believe they receive it and some don't. People who have strong religious convictions in the first place usually find them strengthened when they trust God to provide a good outcome. Others find that their faith wavers, at least temporarily, but almost everyone experiences a test of their religious faith when a tragedy of this magnitude befalls them. The suffering of children has always been a metaphor for doubting the existence of God, but it has also, perhaps ironically, "proved" the existence of a God who creates tests of strength and will.

Psychiatrist

The practice of psychiatry is similar to the practice of any medical specialty in that the practitioner has gone through 4 years of medical school and may have done a few years of general medical residency. He or she then undergoes a psychiatric residency of 4 or 5 years before taking an examination to become board-certified in psychiatry.

The length and complexity of psychiatric training provides a well-grounded basic understanding of all types of mental and emotional function and dysfunction. Fear, grief, and all the other states that families of children with cancer experience are not sicknesses, but if you are seriously depressed and unable to function at your usual level, a psychiatrist may be the best equipped to treat you, especially because he or she can prescribe tranquilizers and antidepressants.

Psychiatrists tend to charge more than other types of mental health counselors, although in major metropolitan areas there is often not much difference between the fees of psychiatrists and clinical psychologists.

Psychologist

A psychologist holds a Ph.D. and provides many of the same services as a psychiatrist, with the exception of prescribing drugs. Psychologists perform many functions (testing, administration, research, and the like), but you will want one who specializes in clinical treatment—that is, working directly with patients both individually and in groups.

Although psychologists tend to see human behavior in terms of healthy or unhealthy characteristics, many, like some psychiatrists, are trained in more nontraditional ways, so you are more likely to find one who will see your feelings as situational problems that have gotten out of hand rather than as symptoms of true mental illness.

Social Worker

A clinical social worker holds a Master of Social Work (M.S.W.) degree and has had training in providing direct patient care. Social workers often do not have the depth of theoretical background that psychiatrists and psychologists do, but most of them have the advantage of seeing life as a series of problems to be solved, and are therefore more likely to see your feelings as situational rather than as pathological. In other words, they're less likely to view you as sick.

Also, many social workers are highly experienced in crisis intervention, that is, helping you compartmentalize your life and deal with the problem at hand—getting through this difficult period—rather than viewing your whole mode of functioning as unhealthy and insisting that you change your entire behavior.

Art Therapist

Art therapy can provide a humanizing influence in the midst of illness, fear, and loneliness. It allows children to be children and to practice developmental skills even during life-threatening physical illness. Tracy Councill of Georgetown University Medical Center says, "Art therapy is used to express feelings in a nonthreatening way, or it can support children's defenses and help them cope with the rigors of treatment."

She describes the benefits of art therapy: reducing symptoms of depression and anxiety; increasing children's sense of control and autonomy; easing communication between the family and health care providers; and providing the child with some effective coping strategies outside the hospital, including relief of pain through distraction.

Art is one of the most potent forms of nonverbal communication. Councill described a 10-year-old boy who rarely talked about his illness and how he felt about it. But when his hair fell out, he saved it and glued it to the wolf in a picture he had painted of a forest. "He gave his hair to an animal associated with strength and control, and he provided a cave to shelter the wolf. In taking care of the animal, he seemed to be taking care of himself and perhaps appropriated some of the wolf's power."

Councill said that she always lets children choose whether or not to participate in art therapy when they come for outpatient therapy. "They have very little choice over anything else that happens in the hospital," she said. Councill prefers not to have parents in the art therapy area. "Parents often have performance goals for their kids," she explained.

"They want the art to be 'good.' They want their children to draw things 'correctly' rather than just let them draw what they feel. Spontaneous pictures can be powerful metaphoric expressions of feelings and beliefs."

Support Groups

Support groups represent another avenue of help that can be used to great advantage by those facing the crisis of childhood cancer. The support group concept was developed 2 or 3 decades ago and has proved so successful that there now seems to be a group for every possible life situation. Groups of families (or siblings or the children themselves) meet regularly to share their experiences. Such groups provide the freedom to express emotions—sometimes strange ones that come as a surprise. One father said, "This is not a social get-together over wine and cheese. In this group, you must have some willingness to stay with the pain and convert it into meaning."

People discuss their feelings of guilt, anger, grief, and fear with others who have had similar experiences. Support groups work because no one can understand what the family of a child with cancer is going through like another family that has experienced the same thing. But groups aren't for everyone. Some people do better if they remain isolated. Some can't share their feelings in a group, and some can't even say the word "cancer."

Support groups not only give the "okay" to be angry but also provide coping strategies and suggest practical ways to get through the experience. The group provides a safe place to "fall apart" for a time, to break down and cry, to not have to maintain a brave exterior for the outside world.

Men and women often react differently to emotional crises, and in some areas there are different groups for husbands and wives.

Leslie Nelson said that organizing support groups for patients is not as easy as one might think. "Children who receive outpatient treatment already come to the hospital two or three times a week (in some cases, every day) for chemotherapy or radiation treatments, and they don't want to make another trip for a group session."

She said that families in which a child has cancer have little enough time to spend together, and the parents are so exhausted and emotionally drained by the experience that she hates to ask them to bring their children to the hospital more often than absolutely necessary.

"Sometimes there are enough kids who live close to one another that we can put them in touch with each other and they can get their own group together."

There are also groups that start as or evolve into more "businesslike" endeavors: providing information and education to the public and to other families; offering practical help and services to members (babysitting cooperatives, transportation); raising funds for small projects (a group newsletter, a social event) or major projects (establishing a fund to pay for treatment for those who cannot afford it); and organizing volunteer activities for treatment centers. One group even started a "wig bank": Children whose hair had grown back after chemotherapy donated their wigs to other children who needed them.

Nelson also said that she and her colleagues have been successful in establishing a "buddy" system—that is, providing each child in treatment with the names of one or two other children their own age who have had similar experiences.

The buddy system provides someone for the child to talk to and do things with—and that someone knows exactly what he or she is going through. There is no substitute, no matter how kind and loving the parent, nor how professionally adept the mental health worker, for the kind of empathy and support that one "buddy" can provide for another.

CHAPTER 8

Adapting and Coping

Parents often are torn between the needs of the sick child and those of their other children. They must also hold down a job and maintain their regular lives in some semblance of order. Sarah said that she had difficulty focusing on anything but the cancer. "Everything else just falls away." She was "lucky," however, because her other children were grown up when her 20-year-old son got leukemia. She also had become accustomed to her husband's emotional distance and had learned not to count on him. She acknowledged that her situation was different from that of most of the other mothers she met. "I don't know how they managed," she said.

People do manage, perhaps because they simply cannot allow everything in their lives to fall apart. If they concentrated just on the sick child, they would alienate their other children and do them irreparable harm. They would also be in danger of losing their jobs and disconnecting from friends and family.

The goal, therefore, is to attend to the sick child while maintaining other aspects of life. Things, of course, will never be the same; there is no hope of that. But this does not mean that life disintegrates. People have an amazing ability to adapt to and cope with the most severe kinds of stress—and to come through the experience not only in good shape, but stronger than they were before.

People cope with crisis on two levels: internal and external. Each level serves a distinct purpose. Internal coping protects the person from psychological disruption and paralyzing anxiety, and it diminishes dis-comfort. External coping represents mastery of a problem in a practical way.

Successful coping entails maintaining self-confidence and emotional equilibrium, as well as reorganizing one's life to accommodate the prob-lem. Coping is not, however, an inborn skill. Coping skills must be learned, and as with any educational process, progress fluctuates from day to day, and there is a good deal of forward and backward motion on the way to successful coping with something as devastating as childhood cancer.

When parents were asked what they thought got them through the experience, their responses had certain characteristics in common: open, honest communication; the support of their spouse and other family members; their child's courage; and trust that their child was getting the most up-to-date medical care available.

Dealing With Hospitalization

In almost all cases, a child will be hospitalized for a while as diagnostic tests are performed and treatment is instituted. Although most hospital stays are relatively short, this is a stressful time for both parents and children, especially coming, as it does, on the heels of shocking news.

Kate, who was 3 years old when she was diagnosed with rhabdomyo-sarcoma, had a younger sister who also required her mother's attention. "I guess my sister got neglected a little," said Kate. "But I remember that on the nights my mother couldn't stay in the hospital with me, she made tapes for me. Some of the recordings were songs that she sang, some were of her reading my favorite books, and some were just stories that she made up."

Kate still remembers how comforted she felt by the sound of her mother's voice in the big, lonely hospital.

Lillian said, "If I could cope with what seemed like the hundreds of people who came in and out of Jimmy's hospital room every day, then I can deal with anything."

She described it as a "cast of thousands," which is what a busy university teaching hospital feels like to most people who have never experienced one. There *are* literally dozens of people who take care of patients, and there are others who work in the institution (and who come into patients' rooms sometimes) but who are not responsible for patient care. "And not one of them ever knocks before barging in," said Lillian.

It is true that little of what one thinks of as ordinary courtesy is practiced in a big, busy hospital, and patients and visitors can be made to feel terribly vulnerable as a parade of strangers march in and out, doing and saying frightening—and often incomprehensible—things.

Parents find themselves telling the same story over and over again—to attending physicians, resident physicians, medical students, nurses, social workers, child life therapists, and practically anyone else who asks. Most people do not like to refuse these repetitions, first, because they believe that each telling is essential to the child's treatment (it is not), and second, because they do not want to alienate the people who are taking care of their child. The apparent lack of communication among various hospital employees is extremely frustrating.

There are, however, ways to combat the feeling that everything is slipping out of control:

- Ask everyone who does anything to or for your child their name and professional function, and what they are doing and why. This gives you information and conveys to the staff that your primary concern is to protect your child.
- Keep a written list of these people. You can't remember them all.
- Find out who your child's primary physician is, and direct all inquiries to him or her. This establishes a continuing relationship and allows that physician to keep track of your participation in your child's treatment and progress.
- If you have questions for the caregivers (and you will), write them down as you think of them. This serves as a memory aid for you, and it will improve your relationship with the doctors. Most of them would rather sit down and answer a list of questions—which will inevitably lead to more questions and a discussion on various lev-

els—than have you ask one or two questions every time you see them. It prevents them from coming to see you as a "pest."

- Spend as much time with your child in the hospital as you can. Mothers and fathers should share overnight visitation.

- Learn as much as you can about treatment procedures. This helps you control your fear and allows you to participate in your child's physical care. That, in turn, will draw you closer to the staff and give you a sense of personally helping your child.

- If you have been asked for the same information a number of times, ask why it is needed yet again. Try to find out what people are asking and why they need to know.

- If you are from out of town, try to arrange housing for yourself before you arrive at the hospital (see Appendix A for sources of help) or call the pediatric oncology social worker before you arrive. Some hospitals, such as the National Institutes of Health in Bethesda, Maryland, contact parents before a child is admitted and help them make temporary living arrangements.

When you feel intimidated by the officiousness of the staff, the aura of hustle-bustle that is almost always present, or the impatience of the doctors and nurses, try to keep the following in mind: even though the reverse may appear to be the case, the entire staff is there to take care of your child. That is its primary purpose. Even though research projects are under way and even though medical students and residents are there to be trained, the *overriding* reason for the existence of any hospital is patient care. *Your* patient. Your child.

Developing a Routine

Routine is what gives structure to our days. It is what helps us get things done and provides a means of planning for the future. Routine also exists so that we can escape from it for a while and act spontaneously— which would be no fun at all if we were not creatures of habit and routine. Routine is what keeps people in control and holds chaos at bay.

Childhood cancer, however, throws routine and control out the window and gives chaos a toehold. Such chaos is not acceptable for the sick child or for the rest of the family. It is important for families to establish a routine, albeit a different one, so that order returns and they feel a sense of control over what is possible to control.

The sick child and his or her needs will come first, of course, at least during the early stages of the illness. However, as soon as the routine of treatment—first in the hospital and then in the outpatient clinic—is established, the family should get together and talk about how they will continue their lives. They must find a way to balance the needs of the sick child, the other children, and the parents. In short, life cannot continue to focus entirely on the cancer.

Children with cancer all say that they want to get back to normal as soon as possible. Many of them would just as soon ignore the whole thing if they could. It is, therefore, not usually the sick child who is the cause of family dysfunction as an aftermath of the illness. The child with cancer wants to be treated "like everyone else" and will be embarrassed and humiliated at being labeled "a kid with cancer" or "a cancer patient."

Although the parents' *tasks* will change temporarily while the child is sick, their parental *roles* will not. The basic parent-child relationship established over the years will not alter, and the more positive that relationship is (loving, firm, kind, helpful, respectful, and so forth), the less difficult the challenge of the cancer experience will be.

It is important, in fact, for parents not to change the way they relate to their child. Doing so, especially easing up on discipline and changing rules of behavior, can send a frightening message to a child: things are far worse than he or she was told. This is also the time for parents to be scrupulously honest about what is happening to the child and what he or she can expect from the treatment.

One of the things that makes routine so comforting is that we do not have to think about why we do things in a certain way. It is routine that saves us from having to make a decision about every little thing we do.

Although it is hard to imagine this in the beginning, caring for a child with cancer will develop into a routine. It must. But in order to establish a routine, parents need to feel confident that they know how to take care of their child. Building such confidence entails the following:

▶ Always know how to reach the child's primary care physician and a nurse at the outpatient clinic. Write the numbers down, post them in a prominent place, and make certain that every member of the family knows how to get medical help in an emergency.

▶ Get an accurate assessment of what your child can and cannot do after discharge from the hospital. Make sure that the entire family has the same understanding.

▶ Learn what precautions have to be taken. For example, must the child be prevented from contact with airborne infections (colds, flu, and the like)? Does he or she need help going up and down stairs? Are there foods that the sick child should not eat?

As time goes on, both parents and children will become very aware of the problems brought on by the cancer. They will also begin to realize which problems will be only temporary and which will be more long-lasting—or permanent. It can, however, be comforting, as well as medically necessary, to have the child tested by a neurologist, a psychologist, or a physiatrist (a specialist in rehabilitation and physical medicine) to find out which deficits will require long-term attention. The sooner such problems are acknowledged and addressed, the better off the child will be in the long run.

Although childhood cancer may be the worst crisis that a person has ever had to face, it is probably not the first one (and for many people, it isn't the worst). It is thus important for people to look back at past problems and try to remember how they coped with them. Which coping skills worked and which did not? Which ones might have been effective at the time but had negative consequences in the long run?

Most people develop adequate coping skills, and when parents look back on the experience, they marvel at how well they got through it. "I thought we were going to fall apart while it was happening," said one father, "but we never did. We just kept going, and doing what we had to—because we had no choice." The literature on childhood cancer reports that most families not only cope well with the illness but are strengthened by it and emerge from the experience closer and more loving than they were before.

It is important to learn to live in the present as much as possible, to take each day as it comes, and to forget about long-range planning, at least for a while. This does not mean ignoring the future completely (there *will* be one); rather, it means focusing on what is happening now and taking each moment as it is.

Although it is more likely than not that the child will survive his or her illness, the possibility of death looms large, especially in the beginning. This is true for the rest of survivors' lives even though as the years pass, the fear loses its grip, which is even more reason for them to get as much pleasure from the present as they can.

Although major family plans may have to be postponed (a trip to Europe or a climbing expedition in the Rocky Mountains), vacations are still possible, as long as they can be fit into the boundaries of a treatment protocol. Weekends away from home are a good way to relieve the day-to-day stress, as are short visits to grandparents and other relatives.

"My parents used to talk about money all the time," said Chris. "They and their friends were always having these little competitions about who could eat in the most expensive restaurant and how much everyone paid for their houses and all that stuff. It was really gross.

"But ever since I got sick, they seem to have shaped up. They don't hang around with a lot of the same people anymore, and we can have as much fun at an Italian deli as at some ritzy place where you have to get all dressed up and be on your best behavior. They're really cool now."

Coping Patterns

According to Chesler and Barbarin (1987), families of a child with cancer develop one or more of the following three coping patterns: 1) being active and assertive, 2) having open family communication, and 3) using a coherent belief system.

Being active does not mean the same thing for all families. Some learn as much as they can about the disease, take a highly active role in caring for the child, and become involved in childhood cancer–related organizations and politics. Others turn to meditation, prayer, and other coping techniques.

Open communication within a family means that feelings and information are shared, and that the truth is told. This style usually spills over into life outside the family, and parents and siblings tell their friends, co-workers, and schoolmates what is happening and ask for support in both tangible and intangible ways. Such people usually expect similar behavior from others and insist on receiving complete information from physicians and other medical staff.

Having a coherent belief system does not necessarily mean one that is grounded in a formal religion, although in this country that is usually the case. Some people lose their belief in God, at least for a time, whereas others find their faith strengthened. The important thing for people who rely on spirituality is to create a sense of order out of the chaotic or random nature of having cancer. It is important to many people that the two questions "Why me?" and "Why my child?" be answered in a manner that makes sense to *them*.

Being a part of a religious congregation is a great help to many people. It provides a place to go for religious, spiritual, and practical help, and it gives an opportunity for members of the congregation to *be* of help.

Relating to Employers and Co-Workers

Although it may seem to parents as though nothing exists besides their child who is sick with cancer, that is of course not true. Parents have to keep their homes running, attend to their other children, and pay their taxes—and someone has to earn a living.

Most people say they find employers and co-workers to be very helpful and supportive during the initial phase of the crisis. Many employers are willing to be flexible about hours and don't dock salary if an employee needs to miss work to attend to his or her child.

Co-workers often pitch in to help. John, a supervisor at a plant that manufactures small appliances, tells about the equipment inspection he was supposed to do every day at the end of his shift. "I had to make sure that all the high-end tools were accounted for and locked up before any of the guys were allowed to leave the plant. It was supposed to cut down on theft, and according to the rules, only a supervisor could do it.

"It's kind of silly because every single person working that area knew what the tools were, and they all can count! So on Monday, Wednesday, and Friday when it was my turn to take Jeffrey to the clinic for his chemo, one of the other guys did the count and the lockup and just signed my name on the end-of-shift report. The bosses never knew about it. We all could have gotten in trouble I suppose, but it was just something you do. I would have done the same thing for any one of those guys."

Some parents say they are less productive at work because they have trouble concentrating, they make more mistakes, and their mind is never fully on the job. Others have the opposite reaction. Sam said, "I feel kind of funny admitting this, but work was the only place where I didn't think about how horrible everything was. I'm an engineer for an aerospace company, and I do very detailed, technical stuff. It has to be perfect. To tell you the truth, I felt lucky to have that kind of job because it was like a little 'vacation' from the stress and tension that we were going through."

Relating to One's Spouse

It is a myth that the stress of childhood cancer splits up marriages, although this does happen sometimes. Husband and wife need to concentrate on continuing to meet each others' needs, and this is difficult, especially in the beginning. But without each other and the security of a safe haven in which it is possible to let down the brave front that one has to maintain around everyone else, the ordeal will be much more difficult than it needs to be.

People need the same things from their spouse after a child's diagnosis as they did before it: loyalty to each other and to the family, a sense of shared commitment and responsibility, mutual respect, and intimacy. A marriage has always been "the most exclusive club in the world" in that husbands and wives share with and entrust to each other thoughts and feelings that no one else is privy to. This does not change when the child falls ill. In fact, many parents say that their marriage becomes their major source of strength during the experience.

Lillian said, "There were many days when I was hurting so badly and the stress was so terrible that all I could think about was getting home, crawling under the covers and feeling my husband's arms around me. There were times when, if I hadn't had that to look forward to, I don't think I could have gone on."

Although it is less common now, many marital relationships have been arranged along gender-specific lines and roles have been clearly defined. For instance, kitchen work belongs to the wife and the yard work is the husband's responsibility. He earns the bread, she bakes it.

These roles will have to change during the child's illness. For example, if the mother spends a good deal of time at the hospital, and the father and other children want to eat dinner, they will have to learn to cook it themselves. They can send out for pizza and Chinese food only so often before it gets boring or too expensive.

Similarly, if the father spends most of his weekend days at the hospital because his work prevents it during the week, and if the hedge and shrubs need trimming and the garbage has to be taken to the city dump, the mother has no choice but to take on these chores.

Many spouses say that these role changes were refreshing after everyone got used to them. Said Sam, "I kind of got into ironing. I still hate the idea of it, but once I get going, I find it relaxing and mindless. It's a good chance to get my thoughts in order—and I do love seeing all those crisp shirts hanging in a row!"

Fighting

Of course, marriages undergo stress during this time. It would not be natural if they did not. Spouses fight and even entertain bitter feelings about each other. Husbands sometimes resent the amount of time that their wives spend with the sick child, and wives get angry about their husbands' inability to express emotion or to seem to care as much as they "ought" to. They also resent having much of the burden of the sick child's needs, as well as those of the household, placed on their shoulders.

The best way to deal with these angry feelings is to set aside time alone to talk about them—that is, to have a fight. If the spouses need to go out of the house to do that, so much the better. Every now and then, all parents need to be away from everything that reminds them of their current situation, and that may mean leaving the sick child alone in the hospital for an evening and hiring a babysitter for the other children.

"Every couple fights," said Brandy Solomon, L.C.S.W., a psychotherapist in private practice in Bethesda, Maryland. "In fact," she added, "learning to fight well strengthens a marriage. A 'good' fight can reinforce respect and mutual caring."

In the course of providing therapy for couples, Solomon has developed a set of guidelines for fighting:

- Don't put off the fight for too long. Anger festers.
- Stick to the current topic, and don't make global complaints ("You always . . . You never . . . ").
- Describe how you feel (use "I" statements), but do not assume that you know how your spouse feels.
- Don't engage in name calling, insulting language, cutting sarcasm, cursing, yelling, casting aspersions on your spouse's family, and the like.
- Ask for what you need and want, but do not blame or accuse your partner if your needs are not met. Stress the positive behavior you would like to see, but don't lean heavily on the negative.
- Accept responsibility for your part in the problem, don't make excuses for your bad behavior, and don't answer your spouse's complaint with one of your own.
- Be an empathetic, active listener, and don't forget that change takes time.
- Appreciate each other's differences and try to realize that nothing is completely black or white, all good or all evil, totally true or totally false.
- Find areas of compromise, and set aside time in the future to determine whether these compromises are working.
- Don't threaten divorce and never threaten physical violence.
- Keep talking. The silent treatment hurts too much.
- If you get too angry, agree to stop for a while and cool off. Don't just walk out of the room and leave the other person feeling rejected.

Ș Never lose your sense of humor, and never fail to see the ridiculous for what it is.

Ș Don't withhold love.

Single Parents

A single parent, especially one who lives far from family and who does not have an adequate support network, faces a true emergency when a child is diagnosed with cancer. Few people have a network that can support a major crisis for a sustained amount of time. Probably the most important source of stress—and one that must be alleviated if the parent hopes to cope successfully—is task overload. Simply put, one parent has to do everything.

Single parents have a particularly difficult time coping with the financial aspects of childhood cancer. Most often, the single parent is the mother. It is still true that in the United States, it is women who lose their jobs first. There are a variety of reasons for this, and it is not within the scope of this book to discuss them, but the fact remains that when a woman suddenly experiences a crisis that will make her work attendance sporadic for a period of time, she is in danger of losing her job.

The new federal Family Leave Act will prevent some of this risk, but it has serious limitations: it applies only to businesses with 50 or more employees, the leave lasts for only 12 weeks, and the leave is unpaid. Therefore, even if a single parent works for a large company and is not in danger of losing her job (at least for the first 12 weeks), she receives no salary for that time, which is probably the worst time in her life to lose income.

But depending on where they live and where their children are receiving treatment, single parents do have avenues of help. The first thing to do is to sit down with a hospital social worker and explain the situation. Of all health professionals, social workers are the ones who are the best equipped to help people solve *practical* problems. They know sources of private, local, state, and federal financial aid, and they are experienced in *getting to* these sources.

Call the insurance company and ask to be assigned a case manager (if the company has not already done this). Most case managers are nurses who also are trained in solving practical problems. They, too, have access to resources—both for the sick child and for other family expenses—that the parent probably did not know existed.

One solution to a financial crisis that may be hard for some people is to ask for help. In the case of a divorced parent, the ex-spouse has to be informed of the diagnosis. Presumably he or she will spring into action for the sake of the child. This is a good time to ask for assistance: with the other children, with finances, and even with the more mundane aspects of life such as doing housework, providing transportation for the sick child to and from the outpatient clinic, babysitting, and the like.

The amount of help, financial or otherwise, that a single parent can ask for and expect from an ex-spouse depends, of course, on the conditions of the divorce and how the former partners feel about each other now. If the spouse who left home has remarried and has children and/or stepchildren, complications may arise.

But regardless of how much time has elapsed since the divorce and what life is like now, the sick child still "belongs" to the parent who left home. That parent still has responsibility for and presumably loves the child. The parents must come together, in some way, for the sake of their child, especially when making treatment decisions.

Most single parents develop relationships with their children that differ markedly from what those relationships were like when the marriage was intact. The children tend to be more adultlike and responsible because they *are* more responsible for things around the house. They develop a greater sense of independence because they have only half a set of parents to lean on. They also may forge an exceptionally close relationship with the parent with whom they live.

Of course, none of this is true in all cases. Some children adapt to divorce in just the opposite way: becoming clingy and babyish, regressing, doing poorly in school, and generally having a hard time with childhood or adolescence. They may not be close to either parent.

There can be other problems as well:

ᴥ Sick children feel guilty that they are now an even greater burden on their parent than they were before the illness.

▪ Siblings have even more responsibility placed on their shoulders, and with that can come anger, resentment, worry, and the fear that the family will totally disintegrate.

▪ The temptation for a single parent to place too much responsibility on an older sibling can be almost impossible to resist, especially if that child is competent and uncomplaining.

▪ The parent may have no one close at hand to provide emotional support, comfort, and a shoulder to cry on. The loneliness of the single state and the grief of a failed marriage or a spouse's death rise to the surface all over again.

▪ Whatever self-confidence the single parent has managed to develop over the months or years since the divorce (or death of the spouse) can evaporate in the face of this seemingly overwhelming new crisis.

▪ Finding adult companionship, let alone developing a loving sexual relationship, becomes increasingly difficult during a child's illness. Lack of such connections can make the parent desperately lonely and depressed.

When childhood cancer strikes, the disruption to the family can be more intense than it is in a traditional family (which, in fact, is no longer so "traditional" in the United States). Single-parent families are now common enough that we all have many such households within our circle of friends and acquaintances. They are as "normal" as the families portrayed by Norman Rockwell, which are still well enshrined in the American fantasy-concept of "family." However, this proliferation of single-parent families has made hospital personnel more understanding of and sympathetic toward the problems of single parents.

CHAPTER 9

Family and Friends

Talking About the Illness

Arthur doesn't tell new friends he has had leukemia because he isn't sure of what their reaction will be. He also thinks he might have been refused a job because of the illness, and when he applied for another one, he decided not to mention it on the application. He subsequently told his supervisor, and there have been no repercussions, but he's not sure he won't be discriminated against again.

He hasn't decided whether to say anything when he applies to law school. He is torn between honesty and pride and trying to prevent people from being unfair to him. He seems genuinely worried about lying, but at the same time he doesn't want to jeopardize his chances of getting into law school because of something that has no bearing on his ability to practice law.

About telling friends that he's had cancer: "The close ones I do because I know it won't make any difference. I haven't told too many new people because I don't want to tell strangers my life story. It's not the kind of thing that comes up in conversation. It's private."

Cordelia doesn't tell new friends either. She finds it difficult to discuss her past illness because it's so personal. She did, however, tell her boyfriend on their first date. "I didn't tell other guys, but I just felt like he should know."

With others she keeps silent. "If I told them, what are they supposed to say? I don't want their pity. It's over. I got through it, and I want to go on to other things."

Has she ever had a bad experience as a result of divulging her illness? Has anyone shunned her after hearing the news?

"No, but I'm pretty selective about who I tell. I don't want everybody to know. The people I tell I'm really close to, and I know they wouldn't run. I guess that's why I choose to tell them."

Joan has had mostly positive experiences when she has chosen to tell others about her illness. "There have been a few creeps in my life, but they are so far outnumbered by the good people that I hardly pay attention to them."

There was one experience, though, that sticks out in her mind. She laughs about it now, but it wasn't funny at the time. "A guy I knew in school—we were just friends—fixed me up with his friend. Actually, the guy had seen me and thought I was cute, but he didn't want to come on to me, so he asked my friend to fix us up.

"We went out on a date, and he kept staring at my head. Finally, he asked if I were wearing a wig and I said I was. He wanted to know why, so I told him.

"He was really cool about it, asked me some questions and said that he thought I was brave to have gone through everything I did.

"The next day, though, he went to where my friend worked and tried to punch him out. He was furious with my friend for fixing him up with someone who had cancer."

Living With Cancer

Over the months of treatment, many children begin to feel isolated from their peers, and they come to see their "real life" as moving farther and farther away from what it had been before they got sick. Developmentally, they regress to some extent. Younger children become more dependent on their parents, and older children may have to move back home after living on their own in a college dormitory or apartment.

A 17-year-old who has had his driver's license for more than a year is going to feel childish and probably resentful when his mother accompanies him to the doctor's office. And a young woman who has just begun to explore the magic of eyeliner and mascara is going to be heartbroken when her hair falls out, and all the eye makeup in the world cannot compensate for the fact that she has to wear a wig.

One of the hardest things that children with cancer experience is having to shuttle back and forth between the world of the sick and the normal world—between being "just one of the crowd" and being a special person who is worried about and doted over.

Growing up means learning new things and finding new ways to relate to people. It means searching for your place in the world and coming to understand what is important and what is not. It means making mistakes and learning from them, and finding out that not everyone thinks the way you do and not everyone's family functions the way yours does.

These are difficult lessons, and most of them have to be relearned over and over again. The process is simultaneously painful and exhilarating. It is both exciting and terribly scary. It involves intense feelings and the joy of discovering new opportunities; it is also stressful and exhausting.

When a child has to combine the task of normal growth and development with the burden of fighting for his or her life, the problems can be overwhelming. There are, however, certain things that all children with cancer seem to need and want:

- Honesty from parents and health care providers
- The ability to confide in a few close people—and the assurance that those people will understand
- Parents who will remain strong for them and who will keep the family functioning as it was before the illness struck
- A positive attitude about survival that is supported and reinforced by family, close friends, and health care providers
- The ability to fight the disease
- A positive self-image, regardless of the physical effects of the disease and its treatment

ᴥ The ability to continue peer relationships, even to the point of having to overcome others' fear of cancer

ᴥ Hope

Above everything else, though, is the need to return as quickly as possible to a normal life. This means curing the cancer, overcoming the side effects, and putting the episode in the past. It does not mean forgetting that the cancer ever happened. That is impossible.

It does, however, mean being able to say, "I had cancer and it was terrible while it was going on, but I'm better now and ready to pursue a normal life." It also means being able to say, "I had cancer, and it was terrible, but I learned many valuable things that I can put to good use for the rest of my life."

Real life, however, is often different from the way things ought to be. If there is one thing that was common to all the young people interviewed, it is the fact that the experience is *never* over. Survivors of childhood cancer may live for years—even for the rest of their lives—as the picture of health, but they can never "get over" the fact that they had cancer as children.

It is with them always, it makes them the people they have become, and they all said that no one, regardless of how empathic or sympathetic, can understand what it is like.

Kate is involved in a career she has always looked forward to: she is a mother. She is happy, healthy (free of cancer for 22 years), productive, and seemingly content. "But I know I have lots of rage bottled up inside me," she said. "Sometimes when my son whines one time too many, or when my husband gets on my nerves, I just snap out and lose my temper, all out of proportion to what is warranted."

She believes that the anger is related to having had cancer and having been left with a serious deformity of her eye and the area immediately around it. "It's mostly because no one else can understand what it's been like all these years—and what it will be like for the rest of my life. People—at least most of them—are kind and nice and try to be polite and helpful. But they can't feel what I feel."

Kate has never participated in a childhood cancer support group and has never had psychotherapy. She says that perhaps when her husband finishes medical school and they have some extra money, she will try therapy. She also acknowledges that a survivors' group probably would be good for her, but it seems unlikely that she will make the effort, for the time being at least.

Friendships Outside the Family

In a study done by Noll, Bukowski, and Davies (1992), popular myths that children with cancer no longer "fit in" with their peers and are cast off as socially unacceptable are shown to be untrue.

Although the long, often painful, and sometimes disfiguring treatment can change children's appearance and deeply affect their moods and view of the world, it is not true that they are stigmatized, teased, and rejected when they return to their peers.

Noll and his colleagues found that children with cancer had just as many friends as their peers, and as many as they did before the illness struck. In addition, they are as accepted for themselves as their peers are for *them*selves. Children with cancer are sometimes slightly more isolated when they return to their usual activities, but that may be because they have missed so much school and perhaps have physical limitations. But these circumstances have no measurable effect on their popularity or friendships.

June found this to be true. She was on chemotherapy for almost 2 years—during fourth and fifth grades—and, for the most part, her friends behaved toward her the way they always had. "Only a few of them knew I was wearing a wig, but no one teased me about it, no one tried to snatch it off my head, nothing like that."

No one knew that June had synovial cell sarcoma, but they did know that she was very ill and taking some pretty serious drugs. Were her playmates exceptionally kind children? "No, I think it was their parents who told them not to ask me questions about what was the matter with me."

Things were not as easygoing in the hospital, however. During the all-day waits in the new pediatric oncology unit, June saw many other children with cancer—or at least what she and her mother surmised was cancer. June refused to have anything to do with any of them. This was in the early 1970s, when there were few established play, art, and psychology programs for children with cancer, so in the waiting room, informal play groups sprang up. "I wouldn't go near any of them," said June. "I was scared of them. They were awful-looking: so sick and sad."

She understands now that she was frightened for herself during those days, that she saw herself in the haggard faces of the other children. But 22 years ago, there was nobody around to gently draw her into their company and to help her talk about her fears.

"I think I'm a more sensitive person now because of that experience," said June. "When I see that someone has a problem or something is bothering a friend, I always ask them if they want to talk about it. I look them straight in the eye and wait for them to tell me what's going on. I try to let them know that I understand what they're going through because I went through bad stuff and I know what it feels like."

All the survivors interviewed describe themselves as being more sensitive toward others. "I grew up having to think about the effect that my illness was having on others," said Kate. "It's a way of life now. I always consider other people before myself."

Extended Family

There are practical considerations when dealing with extended family. The majority of Americans, especially those in metropolitan areas, do not live near their parents, and distance has both advantages and disadvantages. Breaking bad news on the telephone can be either easier or far more difficult, depending on one's relationship with family; physical presence may or may not be a comfort.

"I married fairly late—in my mid-30s," said Marcy, a mother who had lived alone and had devoted most of her energy to her business career before she met her husband. "Steve and I had two kids very soon after the wedding because my biological clock was ticking away, but when Stevie's Wilms' tumor was diagnosed, I dreaded telling my father.

"He always used to blame *me* when I got sick as a child. Even when I was an adult, if I got a cold or the flu, he would ask what I had done to get sick. Didn't I know better than to be in the same room with people who were coughing and sneezing? Why didn't I take better care of myself? That sort of thing.

"So you can imagine how terrified I was to make that phone call. If he always blamed me for my own illnesses, think what a job he could do on me when my kid got deathly sick!"

Marcy never did get the courage to make the phone call. Instead, she explained the cancer in a long letter. "It ended up being a good idea because my dad's memory is not what it once was, and he had this letter to refer to when he needed it."

Marcy's father was used to being waited on by "his" women, so visits from his home in Florida to his daughter and son-in-law in the suburbs of Washington, D.C., were trying. "He never understood why Steve cooked sometimes, and the day that he ran his finger across a windowsill and came up with about 6 months' worth of dust, I just blew!

"My mother was a good housekeeper. She would *never* leave dishes in the sink overnight. But I was so damn tired all the time, and Steve was too. And it just didn't bother me to see unwashed dishes in the morning. Everything got done eventually, but dad wasn't used to thinking of me as less than what my mother would have been—or what he imagined she would have been.

"So I lost my temper and was on the verge of throwing him out of the house when Steve intervened and told him that although we would be glad to see him and have him visit Stevie, that kind of criticism just wasn't acceptable now.

"It all worked out okay because he moved to a hotel in a huff, and I didn't have the energy to deal with his anger and resentment so he had to get over it by himself."

Stevie is in third grade now and in excellent health, but Marcy said that one of the "dozens" of lessons she learned was that she had good judgment in a crisis, and that other people's ideas of the way she handled things didn't matter.

Alan was diagnosed with acute lymphoblastic leukemia (ALL) when he was 2 years old. He was on chemotherapy for 7 years and then had a short period of remission. When he was 9, he was discovered to have a lymphoma and had to begin the treatments all over again.

How does a child survive such a cruel "double whammy"?

"It's 90% mental," said Alan, "and you can quote me on that!"

Alan drew great strength from his family—even though his parents were divorced when he was 5 years old. He is positive that his illness was at least an indirect cause of the breakup. "My dad didn't know how to deal with it. He just wanted to work and drink beer and watch sports on TV. He never talked to me or visited me in the hospital, and he never gave my mom any real help. She was the one who stayed with me and took me to the doctor and fought with the hospitals and got my teachers to come to the house and made sure that I was getting what I needed. She fought for me, my mom!"

When Alan was 12, his mother remarried and had a child with her second husband. "I really think of him as my dad," said Alan of his stepfather, "even though I still see my real father every now and then."

Alan has an older brother and a younger half brother. He feels very close to his family. "When I was little and going through the worst of the treatment for leukemia, my big brother told me that my family would always be there for me. He said that you couldn't depend on anyone else, but you could always depend on your family."

This has remained true for Alan over the years. He speaks of his mother as if she were a saint for the way she took care of him when he was sick, and he voices confidence in the fact that if he is once again visited by cancer (he does not believe that this will happen), his family will be there for him.

Alan lives in a small city in the mountains of Virginia. "Everyone knows everyone else, so my medical history is no secret." This is a source of both comfort and irritation, and it may contribute to his career goals: counseling children with cancer. His major course of study in college (the school is about an hour away from home and he lives in a dorm there) is psychological counseling. When he receives his degree, he plans to get a job in a local hospital working in pediatric oncology. "Then I'll see what I want to do from there. Maybe I'll go on for a master's in psychology, but whatever I do, I know it will involve working with sick children."

Cordelia had both positive and negative experiences with her family during the time she had cancer. She had never talked much with her mother about feelings because her parents are not emotionally demonstrative people. She described them as fairly closed. However, her sister and a few good friends were always willing to listen.

"I really don't think anyone understands, though," she said. "It's lonely, you know. People want to help, but they don't understand what you're going through. The other kids in school didn't have to deal with what I did, and I looked at them as kind of immature. It's not their fault; it's just that my experience was so different."

She said she understood her family's inability to show their feelings, but still, she wished they had been able to talk more. "They all knew about the cancer before I did, and that made me angry. Suddenly, they were all especially nice to me, and that made me feel that something was different."

Cordelia never missed school. She went to the hospital on Friday afternoons for chemotherapy and then recuperated over the weekend from the worst effects. She graduated with her class—and demonstrated her determination to get on with life despite the cancer. She's a junior in college now and plans to be a nurse.

Why does she think she survived Hodgkin's disease when others didn't?

"I was taught never to quit. I think that has a lot to do with it. I don't know what it is. Maybe it's just the way you're brought up. Maybe religion has something to do with it. I don't think you're given anything you can't handle. In my family, everyone works hard. They play hard. They do everything to the best of their ability. Death never occurred to me. The whole time, it never occurred to me that I might die from this. I just endured it and planned to be done with it. I wanted to get over the illness so I'd be able to go on with my life."

Has she been able to do that?

"Yes, I have."

She said this in a positive tone and added that she thinks of herself as cured. She *had* Hodgkin's disease but doesn't have it now. At first she worried that it would come back, but as time passed, she thinks about it less.

Rose said that she would not have been able to "make it through" without the support she received from her family. "My mother stayed with me the whole time I was in the hospital in New York, and even though my father had to go back to North Carolina to work, he was very much with me in spirit. I spoke to him on the phone all the time, and I know he was praying for me."

There was one disturbing thing, though. Early on in her illness, Rose was asleep in her hospital bed—or at least her parents thought she was asleep. Her mother and father were sitting together at the foot of her bed, talking about her. "I heard them say, 'If we lose her, we can't complain because she's been such a wonderful daughter'—or something like that. I don't remember the exact words, and I went right back to sleep, but I remember being very scared at what they were saying."

Rose did not know at the time how very sick she was, and apparently her parents had no idea that people hear things that it's difficult to imagine they can hear. In fact, hearing is the last sense to fade before sleep (or death) closes in.

Siblings and Grandparents

Siblings

Brothers and sisters are angry at the cancer, and they may be furious that their sister or brother is sick. Some of them, however, are better at recognizing these feelings in themselves than their parents are. They may be jealous also, not because they want the disease, but because they're not getting the attention they used to. They're apt to feel left out of the rearranged family constellation in which the sick child is the "bright star." Bluebond-Langner (1978) says, "Siblings of chronically and fatally ill children live in houses of sorrow."

They do indeed. They may not understand that their sibling has a good chance of survival and thus may grieve unnecessarily. Some of them develop problems that are as serious and even more long-lasting than those of the child with cancer.

Factors that influence the way siblings react to childhood cancer include these children's age and maturity, which affects what they are able to understand about the illness; what they have been told about the illness; their relationship to the patient; the way the family has functioned in general, especially in coping with previous crises; and the honesty with which the parents talk about the illness—and about everything else.

Very young children—infants and toddlers—usually have the hardest time when a sibling is diagnosed with cancer because they cannot understand the parents' preoccupation with the sick child and often incorrectly interpret it as rejection of them. Neither do they have the coping skills necessary to adapt to the increased anxiety in the household.

Some sisters and brothers feel stigmatized at school, as if the tragedy in their family were contagious. Young classmates often don't have the words to express the sympathy and concern that they might be feeling, so they say nothing and do nothing, leaving the sibling of the affected child in lonely isolation—hurt and angry. Many siblings feel torn between loyalty to their sick brother or sister and the need to avoid the stigma that the illness causes.

Some siblings feel ashamed at being different from their peers—that is, by having a critically ill child in the family. This is especially true if they have an incomplete understanding of the illness, including the fact that they had nothing to do with it and in no way caused their brother or sister to get sick. The end result of these negative feelings can be school phobia, which, if allowed to continue, can develop into a serious problem.

Just as the sick child sometimes regresses and loses developmental skills, so do many siblings—out of jealousy, fear, confusion, and pain. Younger siblings may wet their beds at night and have nightmares. Their appetites may change drastically, and they may indulge in the kind of temper tantrums that parents thought they had outgrown—or that they had never exhibited before.

Older siblings share the same feelings as younger ones, but they tend to demonstrate them in different ways: psychosomatic illnesses; decreased ability to concentrate, which often results in falling grades in school; sleep disorders; panic attacks about their own health; and even alcohol or drug abuse.

To avoid sibling jealousy and rivalry and to diminish fear and anger, parents should not only pay as much attention as they can to their other children, but also be scrupulously honest with them about what is happening. They might want to enlist the siblings' help in getting through the crisis so that everyone views the family as a team that works together to beat the cancer.

Honesty does not mean a "one-shot" discussion early in the illness with no follow-up talks. Parents need to evaluate from time to time what their children understand. Siblings need to be kept abreast of developments, to be reminded of the facts, and to be given opportunities to ask questions and talk about their feelings.

Children almost never understand completely what their parents have said, especially about important and frightening subjects. Thus, what they "know" about their brother's or sister's illness may turn out to be a combination of fact and fantasy, with the latter often predominant. Misinformation, then, adds to feelings of anxiety, fear, depression, and hopelessness.

Older siblings can participate in family conferences; they can even attend meetings between parents and physicians about the patient's treatment. Younger children should be encouraged to join in the play activities at the hospital and to accompany their siblings on a few trips to the outpatient clinic.

Siblings can provide a tremendous amount of support and encouragement to a sick child. All siblings, especially if they are close in age, form alliances against their parents. They all have secrets they don't share with parents. They get into hot water together and share the burden of guilt. They are a sort of "inner club" within the larger family organization, and it is this closeness, this sense of unity, that can give the sick child the courage and strength to go on with the treatment. The child who dares his kid brother to forbidden thrills is not going to let that brother give up treatment when things get rough.

Karen said that much of her positive attitude came from her sister. "Pam was a major factor in helping me to stop dwelling on the leukemia. There are other things to do and think about, and she helped me to see that—more than she will ever realize."

Kate's sister, who is a year and a half younger than she is, was very protective of her while she was sick. "If kids teased me or made fun of my eye, my sister would be right there, telling them to get lost. She was even ready to fight for me if she had to. She watched over me like a little assistant mother—even though she is younger than I am."

Joan's two older sisters also provided help and support. She was 16 when her leukemia was diagnosed. "After I had been on chemo in the hospital for about a week, and I started to feel a tiny bit better, my middle sister helped me take a shower and wash my hair. She put a little makeup on me, and generally made me feel like a person again."

Joan's brother was only 10 years old when she got sick. "He wasn't allowed to visit me in the hospital because they were afraid of the germs he might bring with him. You know how little kids are always having some kind of communicable disease.

"That made it very hard for him to deal with the illness. He really didn't understand what was happening to me, and I think that because he couldn't come to the hospital to see me, he was the only one in the family who was positive that I was going to die right then."

Joan and her little brother developed a routine that somewhat compensated for his not being able to visit her. "Every night at 9:00 on the dot, he would call me to say good-night. We would talk about things, routine ordinary stuff. But it reassured him that I was still around, still his big sister. That little talk meant a lot to both of us, and I think it started the really close relationship that we have now."

She tells a story of something that happened about 4 or 5 years later. It was when her hair had just started growing back in, and once in a while, she would feel brave enough to go out without her wig. On this day, she took her brother and his girlfriend to a mall.

"I was going to walk around the mall for 2 hours while they went to a movie. After I had left them at the theater, I saw two teenage girls staring at me. They were looking at my head and giggling, and one of them told the other how weird I looked. They said it right out loud, almost as if they wanted me to hear.

"I ran out to the parking lot and sat in the car and cried for an hour and a half. My brother asked me what had happened, and I told him. Then he said something that I had never realized before. He said that he truly understood how I felt, that maybe he was the only one in the family who did."

Joan's brother had been born with a cleft lip and palate, and although he had had corrective surgery, he still had a slight facial deformity and had always been sensitive about it. "I never thought about it," Joan said, "because I was so used to seeing him. But when he made that comment that day in the mall parking lot, that established a bond of closeness between us that I don't have with anyone else in my family."

The visibility of the illness and the treatment can have a powerful effect on the way that siblings react. A "hidden" disease like leukemia or

Hodgkin's can be more frightening and sinister than a more overt one in which the tumor shows. The interior nature of some types of childhood cancer can lead to thoughts such as, "If Beth has this thing and no one knew about it until a few weeks ago, then I could have it too—right now—and no one would know about it."

The fact that this is true, highly unlikely but nevertheless true, makes it much more difficult for parents to cope with—if they indeed hear about these kinds of fears. The fact is that any one of us could be "growing" a cancer at any time. Adults realize this but never think about it because there is nothing that can be done. Children probably didn't realize this before it happened to their brother or sister, but now it might prey on their minds.

Children are highly sensitive to changes in their parents' behavior and feelings. Siblings, too, suffer from separation anxiety, especially the very young ones, because their parents are away from home so often. Parents need to be as open and honest with their children as they can—and as each child's age permits. Tracy Councill tells about a 6-year-old boy who had Wilms' tumor, was treated successfully, but eventually had a relapse and died. His 9-year-old sister was never told what was wrong with him, was never informed that her brother was dying, and was never given the opportunity to share her feelings of loss, grief, and anger.

It is not unrealistic to assume that this little girl will have severe psychological problems that will last well into adulthood.

Parents also must guard against turning older siblings into "little mothers and fathers"—that is, burdening them with the major tasks of running the household while parents are attending to the business of sickness. On the other hand, siblings need to be made to feel that they are an integral part of the family effort to get through the crisis.

Some parents find that their other children eventually become greater and more long-lasting sources of stress than their sick child. If 10-year-old Johnny breaks windows in the neighborhood or shoplifts candy from the local convenience store in order to draw his parents' attention away from his sick brother, the unexpected stress of having to bail a previously well-mannered little boy out of a juvenile detention center will not lead them to offer the kind of attention Johnny craved in the first place.

There are things that parents can do to ensure that the stress of serious illness in the family does not create a negative effect on the sick child's brothers and sisters:

- Make certain that the siblings understand what cancer is and the ultimate effects it might have, especially the fact that it is *not* contagious.

- Try to find out if brothers and sisters believe that they might have been the cause of the illness. Does Susan think that she "gave" her little brother a brain tumor that time last winter when she pushed him off the sled and he bumped his head and cried? How does Tim connect that time 2 years ago when he locked his sister in the hall closet for 2 hours during a thunderstorm when their parents were out—and she was so scared that she wet her pants—with the cancer she now has in her kidney? Children are fantastic dramatists and they have the capacity to create images of horror that would make Stephen King jealous. They are also, depending on their age, not overly proficient in logic. Therefore, parents should never assume that the siblings don't blame themselves for what has happened, regardless of how farfetched such a belief might appear.

- Encourage the sibling to visit the sick child in the hospital as often as possible. Familiarity with the environment of illness will remove some of the strangeness. In addition, it is good for brothers and sisters to see the sick child relating to other sick children—and to see that the pediatric cancer unit is rarely a place of doom and despair.

- Siblings must be made to feel that, although a great deal of their parents' time and energy is being taken up with the sick child, they are still as important as ever—that they are as loved now as they always were, and that their value as human beings and as members of the family has neither increased nor decreased because a brother or sister fell ill.

- Inform the siblings' teachers about what is going on at home. This is just as important as informing the teachers of the sick child.

⋙ Parents need to share their own feelings of anger, sadness, fear, and worry with siblings. If children can see that adults have the same reactions that they do, and that those reactions are normal and "okay," their need to act out in inappropriate ways will be reduced.

⋙ To prevent siblings from feeling that "my brother gets all the good stuff just because he's sick," ask people not to buy presents for the sick child, except perhaps for an occasional small "being-in-the-hospital" toy.

⋙ Use babysitters that the children know and like.

Victor credits his sister with giving him a tremendous amount of emotional support, even though at the time she didn't realize what she was doing. "She was the only one of all the people I knew who behaved the same toward me after I got sick as she did before."

The incident that signaled the way his sister was going to treat him and his illness occurred as he arrived home from the hospital. "I was so weak that I could barely walk from the car to the house," said Victor. He described the household rule regarding television watching: "Whoever got to the TV set first got to pick the channel, and everyone else had to either watch that program or leave. So when I walked into the living room, my sister was watching something on the tube, I don't remember what. I collapsed into a chair and asked her to change the channel. She barely looked at me as she said 'no.' "

Victor was shocked and angry at this reaction. He was feeling sick and exhausted and sorry for himself and thought that he was owed a certain amount of favoritism in view of his illness—and in view of the way his parents had pampered and fretted over him while he was in the hospital. "But Ellen had other ideas. She wasn't going to give an inch."

Now, almost 20 years later, he and his sister are closer than ever (they are only 15 months apart in age), and Victor feels a good deal of anger and hostility toward his parents, who are still overprotective and treat him like a "poor, sick child."

"I love my parents," said Victor, "but sometimes they drive me crazy." He professed his love so many times that his anger at the way they have dealt with his illness all these years soon became apparent.

Ian is one of six children—his mother's baby, 9 years younger than the sibling closest in age. His oldest brothers and sisters were already in college when he was born, and one brother treated Ian a bit like his own child. "When I was a little baby," Ian says, "Mickey used to take me with him shopping or to the mall, and he would tease the girls about having had a 'secret baby.' "

But Ian's relationship with Jack, the brother next to him in age, was not nearly so loving. "He hated me."

Ian's mother explained, "Jack was the baby for 9 years before Ian was born, and he was several years younger than his next-to-oldest. So he was a little spoiled. Then Ian came along and stole his thunder, so of course he was jealous.

"Then when Ian got sick when he was only 3 years old and I had to give him so much of my attention, you can imagine that all hell broke lose with Jack."

"He was terrible to me," said Ian. "Even when I was finished with the treatment (which lasted 3 years), I was weak and tired all the time. He used to call me a wimp and he hated it when Mom made him play with me and watch over me.

"Sometimes when my parents would go out, he would scare me by saying things like, 'We're all alone now—heh, heh, heh.' He never actually physically hurt me, but he sort of used to try to terrorize me and take little pokes and slaps at me."

Ian and Jack have a close, loving relationship now. What changed things?

"I learned to hit back," said Ian. "When I was about 13, I decided to build up my body and started to work out with weights and exercises and stuff. As soon as Jack saw that I was serious about getting into shape, he helped me do things correctly. He sort of took me in hand. And when he hit me and teased me, I gave it right back to him. That's how I made him respect me."

Grandparents

Grandparents who live close by can be either a hindrance or a help. Those who call three times a day, wring their hands in despair, and spread a cloud of doom over the sick child can do enormous amounts of harm. But those who babysit, grocery shop, run errands, and provide a shoulder for their own children to cry on are a valuable resource. Many older people, especially if they have had a variety of life experiences that have taught them how to cope, can call on wisdom and a certain serenity of spirit to help their own children weather the crisis.

An older person's relationship with a grandchild is based almost solely on love. There is far less of the worry and anxiety that accompanies parenthood. Grandparents are supposed to be for fun, for serious and silly presents, for visits to wondrous places, for stories about "the olden days," for leniency as babysitters, and for limitless supplies of hugs.

Grandparents are not a source of discipline. They don't pay the tuition, but they do sometimes buy the rollerblades and 10-speed bikes. They take grandchildren on fishing and camping trips and don't care how dirty the kids get because they don't have to do the laundry.

Grandparents are free to regard their grandchildren as sources of pure pleasure. But when that pleasure turns to the pain of a life-threatening illness, the pain too is pure and piercing to the core. Many cave in under its weight.

As one woman said, "It's not just my grandson who is suffering. It's my own daughter. My baby is suffering because *her* baby is ill. It's a double source of hurt."

Many people, as they pass through middle age, come to accept the natural order of things and become more aware of their own mortality. They expect to die sooner rather than later, and they are fully aware that their days are numbered. This awareness depresses some people, but it gives others a renewed sense of the sweetness of life and the necessity to experience it as fully as possible because the future is limited.

Thus, when a child becomes seriously ill and might die, the reversal of the natural order of things is especially poignant for older people. And when that child belongs to your own child, the irony can be crippling. More than one grandparent has raged at the unfairness and has pleaded with God to take his or her own life if only the grandchild's could be saved.

Grandparents who refuse to accept or acknowledge the cancer can be a burden to their own children, and some even try to interfere in the treatment. As hard as it is, this is the time that parents must set limits with their own parents, as well as with their children, about how the family will deal with the crisis.

Julia's granddaughter was diagnosed with acute lymphoblastic leukemia (ALL) at age 10, and Julia still has not come to grips with her fear, anger, and grief. She also does not seem to realize, or perhaps she doesn't want to say it out loud, that Jill has a life-threatening illness.

"We were thrilled," she said, speaking of herself, her husband, her daughter, and her son-in-law, "when the test results came back and Jill's cells were the best you could have—if you have to have leukemia. Jill went into remission 3 days later."

Does Julia misunderstand the concept of remission? Her granddaughter, 2½ years after diagnosis, is still receiving chemotherapy, so does that mean that Julia is in a state of denial about the seriousness of the illness?

It was hard to tell. Julia is a clinical social worker who has spent several decades working with the families of sick people. Now she works at a state mental hospital and is adept at using the language of mental health professionals. She smiled all the time as she said things like, "You probably think I'm doing a lot of denial and not being realistic about Jill. But I'm so proud of my family, the way they supported each other through this. They have such good coping skills, and they were all *there* for one another."

Julia talked at great length about how her son helped her daughter, how her son-in-law gave extra "quality time" to their other daughter, how Jill was never left alone for a moment while she was in the hospital, how the whole family rallied 'round the sick child.

But Julia never talked about her own feelings. When she was asked direct questions such as, "Weren't you scared?" "You must have felt so awful for your daughter—helpless," she simply slid around to another topic.

She described in detail who drove whom to the hospital on what day. She knows just when her husband brought balloons to Jill in the hospital. She can tell a visitor how many times her son called for news when the doctors were talking to Jill's parents about the diagnosis and prognosis.

But Julia does not know how she feels about any of this. Or does she?

She refused to acknowledge even the possibility of death from ALL. "We always knew that Jill would get over this. I never once thought about her dying."

Not even knowing that leukemia, regardless of its greatly improved survival rate, is a life-threatening and extremely serious illness? She never once feared for Jill's life?

"Not once," said Julia.

Is she being "brave" for herself? Does she believe that her husband and daughter need to see courage and a positive attitude at all times? Does she think that Jill has no idea of how desperately sick she has been? Or is the fear of death so strong that it is simply too much to bear?

CHAPTER 11

Paying for Treatment

Financial Impact

The financial impact of childhood cancer is enormous—even for families who have adequate health insurance. In addition to the cost of the treatment itself (about which more later), there are the ancillary expenses, which can be just as high and in many cases more stress producing. For families living on the edge of financial disaster, the diagnosis of childhood cancer can push them over into acute poverty. The following are some of the "hidden" costs of cancer treatment for children:

- Some people have to travel hundreds of miles to the hospital, which puts wear and tear on the car, and on gasoline credit cards. Even people who live only a few blocks or a few miles from the hospital have to drive there every day, often two or three times a day, and pay for parking.
- Hotels and motels can be prohibitively expensive, and not every city or town has a Ronald McDonald House or a Children's Inn (for families of children receiving treatment at the National Institutes of Health).
- Parents say their phone bills are astronomical because of the long-distance charges that accrue from calling family members and friends and phoning treatment centers in distant cities.
- Young siblings require babysitters when parents are at the hospital with the sick child.

☙ Many people want and need the comfort of group, family, or individual psychotherapy during the crisis. This is expensive and is not fully
paid for by the vast majority of health insurance policies.

☙ Not all school systems have at-home teaching for children who will
not be able to attend school for a time, and hiring private tutors is
expensive.

Like an aging automobile that "nickels and dimes" its owner into the
decision to buy a new one, the "small" expenses of childhood cancer can
be the most difficult to bear. In this case, there is no option to go out
shopping for a new car, no matter how high the monthly payments.
Financial burdens have to be dealt with as they arise.

Donna said that at times, she was more frustrated by the financial
aspects of the cancer than the medical aspects. "I'm not saying that the
treatment was easy on any of us," she explained. "But once Larry started
chemotherapy and we saw him start to improve, we felt more in control.
Really, all we had to do was make sure he got to the clinic for his
treatment.

"I'm not trying to make light of this. It was much more complicated
than that. Larry puked his guts out in the car on the way home, and he
was cranky and horrid a good deal of the time. But we knew that would
pass. This sounds like a terrible thing to say, but we knew that he would
either die or get better, and we simply didn't entertain the thought of
his dying. So he was going to get better, and all he and his father and I
had to do was wait it out.

"Not so with the money aspect. Larry's cancer drained us of every
cent we had. You know, my husband has a good job—he's a midlevel
manager for the federal government, and I went back to work part-time
as soon as Larry was in school most of the time.

"I had lost my original job right away—as soon as I told my boss that I
needed more flexible hours, what with the chemo schedule and doctors'
appointments—and my child being sick and needing me at home. The
bastard said he needed someone he could count on and that was that.

"My husband's boss was not a whole not nicer, but it was the government, so he didn't get fired. What saved him was the willingness of his
co-workers to cover for him and do a lot of his work. Several times they

even lied to the boss for him. They were great!

"But the money—God. It seemed as if every time we turned around, there was another expense that insurance didn't pay for. Take the garage parking in the hospital, for instance. It was five or six bucks every time we went, which in the beginning, was 5 days a week. I asked administration if there was some kind of a monthly pass, but the clerk just looked at me as if I had lost my senses.

"Then there were new clothes for Larry. Most people would never think of this as a medical expense—it certainly wouldn't have occurred to me before I went through it—but Larry lost so much weight in the beginning that he looked like a little scarecrow. It was depressing to see his clothes hanging off him like that. It made him look even sicker than he was. So I went out and bought him some things to wear until he gained his weight back. Naturally, it was winter!"

Donna laughed as she told the story, but it was not a sound of mirth. The bitterness in her voice was hard to ignore, especially as she said, "It'll be years before we get all the bills paid off. Sometimes I think we'll *never* be able to go on vacation again."

And a vacation is what Donna and her husband needed most right then—just the two of them.

Leslie Nelson, a social worker at Georgetown, said that some families feel as though they're supporting two households—their real one at home, and the ancillary one at the hotel or motel (or with relatives, if they're lucky) where they've camped out for the duration of the initial treatment.

"If they had only one car before, they'll either have to get another one or lease one—or spend a fortune on taxis," said Nelson. If one parent needs the car to get to work, the other has to have some form of transportation to get to and from the hospital.

"You know, it used to be that there were all kinds of agencies that would provide volunteers to drive sick people back and forth to hospitals and doctors' offices," said Nelson. "Of course, the volunteers were mostly women, and that source of help has dried up now because most of those women have gone back to work."

Hospital billing systems can be one of the most frustrating parts of the entire cancer experience. They are often fragmented, there are almost always mistakes on the bill, and the bill itself might as well be written in hieroglyphics for all the good it does to help families understand what was "purchased" for the child, what was covered by insurance, and what has to be paid for out of pocket.

It takes a person of extraordinary patience and perseverance to, first, demand a fully itemized hospital bill and, second, interpret it. Most people find it far too daunting to go over each bill with a fine-tooth comb, so they simply pay whatever the hospital demands.

Leona paid attention to the charges and argued with the hospital, but the process reduced her to tears. "When the bill came, it had things like 'pharmacy services' and 'operating room.' The insurance had paid for 80% of the total, but what was left for us to pay was several thousand dollars, so I wanted to know exactly what I was being billed for. For instance, what exactly did 'supplies' include?

"I called the billing department and asked for more detail, but they never sent it and in a month I got a bill that said SECOND NOTICE in big red letters. That, of course, makes me the bad guy. So I wrote a letter to the director of accounting—first I had to call and find out his name—and said that I'd be happy to pay the bill if I knew what I was paying for.

"Several weeks later, I got what I wanted, but not before the original bill came around again, this time with the big red words SERIOUSLY DELINQUENT on it.

"I had no idea what three-quarters of the things on the itemized bill meant, but luckily my next-door neighbor is a nurse and she helped me with some of it. Together, we found tons of mistakes—stuff we were billed for that Sally never received. I highlighted them all in yellow and wrote back and told the director of accounting to send me a corrected bill. That, of course, took weeks, and in the meantime, the original bill kept arriving every month—after a while with threats of legal action.

"It took 6 whole months to get it all straightened out, but in the end, I got the total cut about in half—that's the amount of mistakes the hospital had made. I'm not at all sure that some of them were totally innocent."

Leona is still angry about what she had to go through with just that one bill. "And that doesn't even take into account the bills we got from the many different doctors who saw Sally—the anesthesiologist, the physical therapists, and all the rest."

Very few people have the time, energy, inclination, or knowledge to do what Leona did about her hospital bill, and thus end up even angrier because they suspect they have been ripped off but cannot prove it. Such experiences add to people's distrust of hospitals and of the health care system in general.

Insurance

One of the first things that parents must do as soon as they have recovered somewhat from the initial shock of the diagnosis is to figure out how they are going to pay for the treatment. Almost no one reads the fine print of a health insurance policy that may have been in effect for years. Moreover, the terms of the original policy may have changed. Fewer conditions may be covered than the policyholder had thought. Some illnesses fall under the rubric of "preexisting condition," and although a new diagnosis of childhood cancer is not one of those, there are insurance companies that will do their best to avoid paying future claims.

On the other hand, some insurance carriers have become more enlightened in recent years and treat childhood cancer as a long-term health problem. They assign specially trained employees—known as case managers—to work with families to provide good treatment at the least expense to both the family and the insurance company. A family that has private health insurance should contact the company immediately and request a meeting with a case manager.

With some large companies, such a request is not necessary because as soon as the claims department receives the first bills for the illness, an automatic computer program alerts the claims staff to the fact that this condition will be expensive and of long duration. Automatic referral is made to a case manager, who will then contact the family.

The whole matter of health insurance can be terribly confusing and frustrating, especially now that it has been so much in the news. There are several different types of health insurance:

- Fee-for-service insurance, sometimes called traditional or conventional plan health insurance, is based on payment (either directly to the insurance carrier or indirectly through an employer) of a certain premium, for which some portion of health care expenses are reimbursed. The size of that portion and the type of expenses reimbursed vary widely depending on the plan purchased, which of course varies with premium price. In a fee-for-service plan, the provider (the doctor or the hospital) first bills the insurance company and then bills the patient for whatever is not covered.

- Health maintenance organizations (HMOs) are types of managed care health insurance plans that an individual or family joins as a dues-paying member—that is, for a flat monthly or quarterly fee (which tends to rise as the organization's expenses increase). The member receives almost all health care at no additional cost. Some HMOs charge a small per-visit fee in order to discourage unnecessary trips to the doctor, and this practice will become more common in the future.

- Medicare is a federal program, enacted by an amendment to the Social Security Act, that provides hospital and medical care coverage for people 65 years of age and older, as well as for some individuals who have been disabled for more than 24 months—including children with cancer. Medicare is not charity, any more than are Social Security benefits. It is a government entitlement program that is designed to cover very basic health care services, such as hospitalization, skilled nursing, diagnostic tests, emergency care, and some durable medical equipment such as wheelchairs, walkers, and crutches.

- Medicaid is a joint federal-state program, also created by the Social Security Act, that provides health services to people who live at or below the federal poverty level and have no other way to pay for health care. Eligibility requirements and services provided vary from state to state.

One of the most painful surprises in dealing with an insurance company is finding out that a child's illness is considered a preexisting condition. This can happen if the cancer was diagnosed before the insurance coverage became effective—for instance, if a parent has started a new job and the employer-provided health insurance does not kick in until 3 or 6 months later.

Some companies will never cover a preexisting condition (which makes it difficult for many adult survivors to obtain health insurance); others will cover the condition after a year has passed since the time of diagnosis—a serious hardship when dealing with childhood cancer, for which the biggest medical expenses occur in the first year.

When a child participates in a clinical trial, the drug or other treatment being tested is provided free of charge. However, other aspects of care often are not paid for by the agency conducting the research. These ancillary expenses are usually not covered by insurance, but people who insist on taking the denial of a claim to a supervisory level at the insurance company often find satisfaction.

Make certain that you find out exactly what the research protocol does and does not pay for (see Chapter 14 for a discussion of clinical research). Ask other parents what their experience and problems with insurance companies have been.

If a treatment is new but not technically experimental, some insurers will balk at paying for it. If the company denies the claim, question that denial. You have been paying premiums for years; now is the time to reap all the benefits. An insurance policy is a legal contract that the company is required to abide by.

If you feel that you have been treated unfairly by your insurance company, complain. If you are insured by a private company or a private HMO, the agency to contact is the state department of insurance, usually in the state capital. If you have been discriminated against by an employer or a union (not the insurer), contact the U.S. Department of Labor, Office of Pension and Welfare Benefits.

If Medicaid is the offender, complain to your state department of social services, and if Medicare or other Social Security benefits are at fault, write to the U.S. Social Security Administration. If you are eligible for veterans' benefits and are insured by the Civilian Health and Medical Programs of the Uniformed Services (CHAMPUS), contact the Department of Veterans Affairs.

All the appropriate addresses and phone numbers are in the blue pages of your local telephone book. Other sources of help and information about insurance matters are listed in Appendix A.

Locating Other Resources

Social workers at children's cancer centers (as well as at general hospitals) are probably the best source of information about financial help available from a wide variety of agencies, associations, and foundations. They also have had vast experience in helping families cope with the financial burdens of the illness.

After learning the diagnosis, finding out what treatment will be necessary, and determining what part of the treatment expenses is covered, a family can restructure its budget and spending priorities to take the cancer into account. Such budgeting decisions are difficult and painful, and may involve "penalizing" siblings. For instance, if money is going to be tight, dancing and baton-twirling lessons become luxuries that will have to be canceled or postponed.

The mortgage or rent has to be paid, the house has to be heated and lit, and there must be food on the table. Outstanding debts—for example, credit card expenses and the car loan—may have to be refinanced, and making such arrangements is never pleasant. Parents will have to estimate the "incidental" expenses of the illness each month (this is where the experience of others is valuable), and then they must decide what activities will have to be temporarily halted to pay these expenses.

On the other hand, no one ought to forgo pleasure altogether. That would be a mistake in many ways. Low-budget recreation can be substituted for more expensive varieties—for example:

- Video rentals and homemade popcorn instead of dinner out and a movie at the theater
- A picnic made at home and eaten in a state park instead of a 2-day trip to a theme park

- Cheap seats on the lawn for the summer concerts instead of the expensive ones in the orchestra section
- Local day trips interspersed throughout the year instead of a winter ski vacation in Colorado
- Clothes shopping in discount stores instead of department stores

Don't forget the deductions for medical expenses to which you are entitled on your federal income tax. Keep track of all incidental expenses, because you are entitled to claim many of them, such as travel expenses to and from visits to health care providers, out-of-pocket costs for prescription drugs and medical equipment, and even meals during long stays. For example, if you have to travel out of town with your child for treatment, some or all of your hotel room and meals are deductible. Ask the Internal Revenue Service or your accountant for details, but *do* take every penny of deductions to which you are entitled.

CHAPTER 12

School

The vast majority of children with cancer (more than 80%) experience disruptions in their academic career. Some miss only a minimum amount of time, which they make up with home teaching, whereas others miss so much school that they end up being held back a year.

School and the friends made there, as well as the activities that school provides, make up a child's entire social life. In fact, school is one of the primary influences on his or her life. School is where children learn to work together cooperatively (team sports and academic projects), and friendships formed there last for years, sometimes even a lifetime. Children learn how they are perceived by others, and they refine their sense of how their actions affect others.

Even more important, school is practice for the future. It teaches self-discipline, reinforces the concept of reward for work well done (and punishment for slacking off), and introduces some of the exterior controls that the world imposes on all of us.

Anything that significantly interferes with school can seriously affect the child's entire life. About half of children with cancer (54%) reported disruptions in their peer relationships and decreases in extracurricular activities. Almost half (46%) said they changed their future academic plans because of the cancer, and 38% changed their career plans. More than 25% said they experienced academic difficulties after they returned to school.

Some adolescents say they feel that their academic performance improved when they returned to school because they felt a greater seriousness of purpose, more self-confidence, and an increased sense of commitment to doing well.

They also reported feeling differently about some of their friends. As one girl said, "The ones who stuck by me, I feel even better about. I feel as if they are *really* my friends. The others—well, the heck with them. I don't have any use anymore for 'fair weather' friends."

Some children make an effort to teach their peers about cancer. They try to bring their classmates to an understanding that they are the same people they were before they got sick. But just as their values about many things changed with the experience of coming close to death, so do their values about friendship. As Cynthia said, "You're either my friend and you care about me for myself, or I don't want you in my life."

School friendships can be a source of comfort and support for children with cancer. A best friend or two can stick up for the sick child if teasing starts to hurt, and friends can explain to other children what is wrong with Mary and why she "looks so funny."

Friends' parents can be more of a problem than the peers themselves. Despite a vastly improved level of knowledge about health in general, there are still many myths and a widespread lack of accurate knowledge about cancer. Many people still believe it is contagious, and parents instruct their children to stay away from their friend with cancer. There is also a belief that involvement with a child who might die would be too negatively stressful for children. This is untrue. The guilt that healthy children experience at abandoning a friend will far outweigh the sadness of seeing that friend in the hospital—or in a coffin.

The only way to combat these hurtful experiences is for the parents to get together to talk about their children's friendship.

"Every time Leah went over to her friend Susan's house to play, the kid's mother came to the door and said that Susan was busy or doing her homework. There was always some excuse. The woman never asked Leah to come inside—as if her leukemia would contaminate the whole house. I was furious. These two kids had been inseparable since they were toddlers."

This mother fumed for a while and tried her best to comfort her daughter. "But how do you explain betrayal to an 8-year-old?" Finally, she and her husband invited the parents to dinner one evening. Leah's mother explained what leukemia was and gave her some pamphlets that she had found at the hospital.

"When Leah came into the dining room and kissed us good night, I could see that woman cringe, but her husband saved the day. 'How about a kiss for Susie's father?' he said. I could have hugged him myself."

Leah and Susan play together now, but Leah still isn't allowed inside her friend's house—unless the father is home.

School officials, even nurses who work at the school, are often just as ignorant about childhood cancer as anyone else, and although it seems unfair, it usually falls on the parents to explain to teachers and school administrators what the child does or does not need.

Sometimes a hospital nurse or physician will contact the school, but this is not the usual practice. The responsibility once again falls onto the parents' shoulders, and many simply don't think of it, or are too tired to deal with it—or don't realize the necessity of "teaching" teachers about childhood cancer.

In such cases, it is only when the child's performance begins to decline, or when he or she gets a serious case of school phobia, that parents realize that something needs to be done.

On the other hand, there are parents who make unrealistic demands on the school, treating teachers and administrators as if they were "junior doctors." The school nurse is the only one who has had health-related training, and even he or she is not equipped to do more than provide emergency medical care. The nurse should, however, be prepared to act as a liaison between a sick child and his or her various spheres of life: home, the classroom, and the hospital. This means that the nurse is responsible for conferring with parents, teachers, and school administrators, as well as hospital personnel, about the child's special needs. Again, although it seems as if this should not have to be the parents' responsibility, it is often up to them to make the initial contact with the school nurse.

The national rate of absenteeism from school averages 3%, but 53% of children with cancer miss some school days during the first year after diagnosis. That rate drops steadily (to 14% in the third year), but being absent this much creates serious problems: trouble getting along with classmates, less inclination to participate in social activities, increased shyness, diminished ability to concentrate in class, feelings of isolation and loneliness, self-consciousness about physical impairments, and resultant depression.

Even when children with cancer attend school, they may not be fully there because they are tired, perhaps nauseated, and may have problems with mobility. Parents worry about their child's exposure to the many infectious diseases that lurk in school hallways, and major outbreaks of measles, chicken pox, or other communicable diseases are a serious source of concern.

Returning to School

Planning the child's return to school is crucial. It should start right from the beginning of the illness. Although school may be the last thing on parents' minds during the early days of treatment, it remains front and center in the child's mind.

Cynthia said, "All I could think about was what the other kids were doing in school. I was just starting to get the hang of that stupid algebra stuff, and I worried that I'd forget it and have to repeat eighth grade when all my friends were starting high school.

"And I had these braces on my teeth, and I was terrified that they'd have to be taken off and that I'd have buck teeth for the rest of my life. I knew my hair would grow back, and it's not that I *liked* being bald, but the other kids in the hospital said your hair grows back and I believed them. But I thought that my teeth would be stuck that way forever."

Cynthia's parents were terrified that she would die, and she agonized over algebra problems and buck teeth.

The earlier the child returns to school and the fewer days of class he or she misses, the easier the reintegration process is. The social and academic ramifications of missing school are minimized if not much time has been lost in the first place. In fact, it is vitally important that the child return to school quickly and continue to participate as fully as possible in all his or her usual activities.

There are things that parents and school officials can do to make returning to school easier:

- From the outset, even during the initial phases of hospital treatment, have the child maintain contact with one or two close school friends. This keeps the school bond tight, and it provides an opportunity for the friends to see that cancer, although frightening, can be dealt with and is not an automatic death sentence.
- Suggest ways that the child can explain to classmates what has happened: perhaps a "show and tell" demonstration with a doctor and nurse as classroom guests—or a science project that can turn personal misfortune into academic achievement.
- Role-play with the child to anticipate questions that schoolmates might ask:

  - How come you're bald? Is your hair ever going to grow back?
  - How does the artificial leg connect to your stump?
  - Can I see your scar?
  - What did it feel like when they were zapping you with those rays?
  - How're you going to get it up if you don't have two balls?
  - Are you always going to look like that?
  - What's that funny thing on your lip?

- Encourage the child to attend school as much as possible. Set limits for what constitutes a "legitimate" excuse for staying home.
- Ask the child's brothers and sisters to help with the return to school by explaining to classmates what has happened and why their sibling is not to be feared, shied away from, or taunted because of the cancer.
- Make certain that school officials and teachers understand the effects of the disease and the treatment that might cause irregular attendance, fatigue, learning disabilities, and self-consciousness about physical disabilities. This requires a conscientious effort on the part of the parents (who are the primary advocates for the child) as well as the educational system and health care providers.

- Join parents' groups that inform the educational community about the effects of childhood cancer and that act as advocates for children.

- Make certain that school officials and teachers have current medical information about childhood cancer and that they are not burdened with myths, superstitions, and negative attitudes—or, if they are, that they don't use those attitudes to harm or discriminate against the child.

- Establish a "happy medium" between overprotectiveness and sufficient protection from vulnerability. This is not easy, but it is the parents' responsibility to set the tone for teachers and school officials regarding how their child is to be treated.

- Find out what school policies will affect the child. For example, if wearing a hat inside the school building is prohibited, and your child won't wear a wig, ask if the rule may be relaxed just until his or her hair grows back.

Ideally, school reentry should be managed by a team of educational and health care professionals, but this is often not the case. Not all hospital social work departments are equipped—nor do they have the time or inclination—to interact with teachers and principals to establish a special curriculum or program for a child with cancer. Not all doctors and nurses will go to the child's classroom and instruct the teachers and the other children about cancer. Not all teachers are quick to recognize that learning and behavior problems may be the result of the disease, not that the child is stupid or has poor manners. And not all schoolchildren are kind to and understanding of the different one in their midst.

We live in a far-from-ideal world. Therefore, parents need to be assertive in smoothing the way for their child at school. They must be the ones to instill a sense of responsibility in the child and insist that he or she not be excused from meeting all academic requirements just because of the cancer. Parents will probably have to go to school—more than a few times—to meet with teachers, administrators, and ancillary personnel (the school nurse, psychologist, and physical education teacher, for example) to ensure that the child is performing adequately and is receiving any and all special help and adjustments available. They may have to insist if the school balks at fulfilling its responsibility.

Age Makes a Difference

Elementary school and high school children have similarities and differences in the way they react to returning to school. Both groups are concerned about body image, but peer pressure to conform and to "be like everybody else" increases as children progress through high school. Elementary school children are more likely to accept physical differences and handicaps because they see them as something special and unique—not necessarily a negative characteristic.

High school students interact with more teachers and greater numbers of students. There is more intermixing among grade levels, and mobility becomes a problem because students move from classroom to classroom for different subjects instead of staying in one place most of the day, as elementary school children do.

The greatest obstacle to returning to school is the child's fears of classmates' reactions. This anxiety is often justified, because children can be incredibly cruel to each other.

Rose told a story that was horrifying in its simplicity and insensitivity. She spent her senior year at boarding school on chemotherapy, and of course her hair fell out.

"For some reason I didn't want people to know I was wearing a wig," Rose explained. "My roommate knew, and even though she was real good about keeping secrets, somehow a rumor got started that *someone* in my class was bald and wore a wig. I knew about the rumor, but I just didn't feel like telling anyone that it was me.

"One day in the dorm, this girl came up to me in the hall and stared at my head real hard. I knew what she was doing, and I was just getting ready to walk on by when she reached out and sort of knocked my wig off center. She moved it just enough to satisfy herself that I was the one."

Rose was so shocked at this cruelty that she didn't know what to do. "I just stood there. I was so surprised that I couldn't say anything. I don't even remember if I cried right in front of her or if I waited until I got back to my room."

Children also are uncertain about how much to tell their parents. Brian tells this story: "Once when I was a little kid [he's 11 now], two big boys beat me up and stole my baseball glove. When my mom asked who gave me the black eye, I told. She reported the kids to *their* moms, and then one day they were waiting for me when I got off the school bus and beat the s__t out of me because I was a tattletale."

Brian had no desire to repeat *that* experience, but when the teasing at school about the way he looked became too much to bear, he wanted to tell his mother. He solved the problem by asking his mother for help but refusing to name names. His mother went to school and demanded that the harassment stop—and it did. "I know that at least one of his teachers gave the kids a little talking to about tolerance, but Brian himself did the best job," said his mother. "He punched a little boy in the stomach. The kid must have been off balance anyway because he went down in a heap, and everyone assumed that Brian wasn't as weak as he looked. It was a lucky punch, and Brian and I are both sure he could never do it again, but neither of us is telling!"

Children *can* be cruel, but most often they don't want to be. Much of the teasing and shunning arises not from malice, but from not knowing how to behave or what to do. Do you talk about the illness or ignore it? Either route is fraught with uncertainty and the fear of making a mistake. It is easier for some children to ignore the issue—and thus the sick child.

Adolescents have the most to lose if school reentry and continuing experiences are not good. Competition for college acceptance is fierce, and anything that puts a high school student at a disadvantage can have lasting effects. Unfortunately, many college admissions offices, especially in big universities that receive thousands of applications each year, do not look much beyond grade point average and performance on scholastic aptitude tests to determine suitability for admission. This is probably not fair, nor is it necessarily a good way to predict who will do well in college, but it is a fact of life, and parents and children need to accept the reality.

High school students who do not plan to go to college face a job market that becomes increasingly competitive each year. Those who have done well in school and perform well on various vocational aptitude tests get the best jobs—and thus have the best preparation for going on to college later if they choose.

If, for some reason, the child cannot go back to school, or if he or she will have frequent absences, the parents must arrange for academic lessons to continue at home or in the hospital. There are two main reasons for this: First, eventually the child will return to school, and it is important that he or she reenters the same grade and knows approximately the same material that classmates know. Second, and perhaps more important, to stop a child's educational progress gives him or her a subliminal message that there is no future. All parents want their children to do well in school, and all engage in some type of nagging or prodding about homework and grades. This, of course, will stop short when the child falls ill, but as recovery progresses and life returns to normal, an absence of the usual concern about schoolwork will signal its lack of importance.

"Why should this be so?" the child will ask himself. "If school isn't important anymore, maybe things aren't as okay as they say. Maybe I really *am* going to die, and they're too chicken to tell me."

Educational Rights

Two major laws protect the rights of children with cancer who may have learning disabilities and/or various physical limitations. The laws are federally mandated, but the authority to implement them belongs to state governments, which usually allow local school districts to implement the laws.

The federal Education for All Handicapped Law (PL94-142) requires states to provide a free and appropriate education in the least restrictive environment for all handicapped individuals between the ages of 3 and 21 years. The law also mandates the development of an individual education plan (IEP) for each child and requires that both regular and special educators receive training about handicaps.

Although not all children with cancer have disabilities, many do. In fact, PL94-142 specifically covers children with cancer. Therefore, it behooves parents to understand the eligibility requirements and to insist that school districts comply with them. The school district is responsible for evaluating a child's handicap and for providing the necessary services; however, some administrators are more resistant than others, and some do not want to believe that cancer is a "handicap" in the usual sense. It is thus up to the parents to act as advocates for their child.

The law also provides for the education of children who cannot get to school. Most large pediatric units have hospital-based teachers who conduct formal classes for at least a few hours a day, either in groups or on a one-to-one basis.

Homebound teachers are provided by public school systems as long as a physician signs a certificate of need. In some school districts, the actual physical presence of a teacher is supplemented by teaching via telephone hookup, closed-circuit television, and various computer programs.

The Rehabilitation Act of 1973 (PL93-112, Section 504) prohibits discrimination against handicapped people by any federally supported entity, which includes all institutions of higher education that receive federal funds—that is, any large college or university. The law upholds the right of students to receive the services they need to attend school safely and successfully even if they do not qualify for special education. This means that a qualified handicapped person cannot be denied the opportunity to participate in or obtain any of the programs or services offered to any other enrolled student.

Although the law does not specifically address the issue of discrimination in the application process, it seems reasonable to assume that a high school student who has been denied admission to a college or university because he or she has had cancer could make a legitimate case against the school, as long as the student could show that the school would have granted acceptance absent the student's history of cancer.

CHAPTER 13

The Long Haul

Having had cancer means that one is different. Most of the survivors interviewed for this book said they thought they were more mature than their peers, that they had grown up faster. Although many said there *is* some loneliness involved in being different, none said it was altogether a negative experience.

Feeling different from one's friends can be dealt with, but coping strategies have to be learned. Children with cancer must be taught how to recognize and understand what works for them and what does not.

Newfound confidence (without arrogance) is the characteristic that one sees most often in survivors of childhood cancer. Most said they would go through the treatment again, even the ones who had had the worst experiences. "If I beat it once, I can beat it again," is the predominant attitude.

These survivors reported that their values and priorities had changed. Several said they no longer got upset or depressed over "little" things, and they all seem to have a new appreciation of life—that is, of simply being alive, or, as Arthur put it, "being able to walk around and enjoy the blue sky."

In many respects, the success of cancer treatment can be measured as much by the way the child reenters normal life as by the results of blood tests and biopsies. This is because cancer is far more than a wildly malignant proliferation of a group of cells. It is a life-altering disease.

The vast majority of children who survive cancer do so in a manner that suggests that having had the illness was a positive (if not desirable) experience.

Karen expressed it well: "I just got a new Honda and if I smash it up, so what? It's only a piece of machinery."

She said this not in a cavalier manner or to indicate that she has no respect for property. Rather, she meant that she knows what's important and that, when comparing the value of a new car with that of being healthy, there's no contest. She says she feels sorry for people who have never learned to make these distinctions.

She rents a carriage house on the grounds of a large estate. The feeling of peace and relaxation in that little house was almost over-whelming. Some of it had to do with the bucolic setting, but most of it was because of Karen herself. She is a woman at peace.

She doesn't have everything (or everyone) she wants, but she takes obvious pleasure in what she does have: friends, family, her job, and her cat Reggie.

"I've never stopped doing what I want. When I was going through a lot of pain, it might have hurt, but I've never not done anything. My parents never told me that I couldn't do this or that. Sometimes my mom is a little overbearing about wanting to protect me—even now, but we can always talk about it. My family is *very* close."

Rose says that the cancer is "behind" her now. "For a long time after I stopped treatment, it was right there—in my face. I thought about it all the time, I worried about it coming back. It was just *there*.

"Then I learned to let go of it a little. The knowledge that I had had cancer was still with me, very much part of my life, but it didn't seem to affect everything I did. It was like it was sort of walking beside me, keeping me company but not interfering.

"Now it's behind me. It's there, of course, it will always be there because it's something that happened. But I'm past it now. I feel like I can slow down and live more normally."

Rose said that for about 15 years after her treatment ended, she felt as though her life were on "fast forward." She needed to do everything she wanted to do as soon as possible in case the cancer returned. "I went around trying to be all things to all people, taking care of everyone but myself. I felt as though I were holding my breath, waiting for it to come back."

When the cancer was 17 years behind her, Rose discovered a lump in her abdomen. At first she panicked, but the lump went away shortly thereafter and she thought no more about it. "But when it came back, I forced myself to go to the doctor and get it taken care of right away—not like the first time."

The lump turned out to be nothing, just a benign tumor, but it had to be removed surgically and Rose once again spent time in the hospital. "This time, I decided to set some limits and take care of myself. When I was convalescing, I let people know that I got tired easily, and I said 'no' when people wanted to come and visit me. It's just too exhausting to play hostess when you're sick."

Rose said that the second hospitalization taught her a big lesson. "Before the surgery, when I thought the cancer had come back, I thought about my life and all the things that I had done, and I thought that if I was going to die, it would be okay."

Rose didn't *want* to die, but she was no longer afraid of death. She realized that she had had a good life, despite having had cancer—perhaps *because of* having had it—and she was grateful for the support that her family provided and all the good things that had happened to her.

"All of a sudden, I felt as though it would be okay to relax, that I didn't need to do everything as fast as I had been," she said. Even when the biopsy came back negative and Rose recovered from the surgery, she didn't fall back into the frenetic lifestyle that she had adopted as a result of the cancer. Life is still good; it's just slower now.

Survival should be considered a *process* rather than a phenomenon in itself. That is, all of us "survive" life until the moment of our death. In the same way, we might say that a child has survived cancer from the moment of diagnosis until the moment of his or her death—regardless of whether that death occurs a year after the diagnosis or at a ripe old age. The act of surviving is distinguished by how life is lived after the diagnosis, not just by the fact that one has managed to avoid a second or third bout of the disease.

This, however, is a relatively existential way of looking at survival.

There are practical tasks at hand, and now that more children who get cancer are surviving to adulthood, research is beginning to show how they have managed to incorporate the fact of having had cancer into the rest of their lives—how they approach the present and the future.

The Candlelighters Childhood Cancer Foundation recently conducted a survey of children between the ages of 14 and 29 years who had survived cancer. Although the results of this survey might be somewhat skewed because not all of the survivors who received the questionnaire responded to it, the vast majority of those who responded agreed that although they felt different from others of their age who had not had cancer, those differences were positive.

The most frequent difference reported was that the survivors felt more advanced or more mature in their personality and psychological development.

A second positive difference was that these survivors believed that they knew more about the purpose of life. They were able to find meaning in everyday activities and encounters, as well as engage in long-range planning. In other words, although they planned on having a future, they didn't sacrifice present pleasure.

The third most common difference that the survivors experienced was a negative one: physical limitations and a feeling of being weaker and less healthy than their peers. This, however, should not necessarily be interpreted as an entirely adverse phenomenon. Acknowledging physical differences, even significant handicaps, can reflect a realistic attitude and become both a positive coping strategy and a route to increased self-esteem.

The "upbeat" outlook of many survivors of childhood cancer should not be regarded as a Pollyannaish philosophy of ignoring anything unpleasant or painful. Rather, it should be seen as reflective of a sense of self, of newfound strength, and of the discovery of workable coping mechanisms.

If these young people sometimes hide their fears and insecurities from their caregivers, their families, and even themselves, it may be as a result of their need to protect others and, in the process, bolster their own flagging self-confidence. These survivors have been engaged in a struggle for their very lives, and they have emotional and physical scars to show for it. But if they present a positive outlook to the world and adopt an optimistic manner, they establish positive expectations from others that will rub off on themselves. To say to the world, "I don't want or need your pity," is to say to oneself, "I am not a person to be pitied."

In a sense, survivors of childhood cancer are *not* different from the rest of us. There is not a person alive who has not faced a difficult hurdle or come face to face with tragedy, paralyzing fear, or death. Everyone faces tests of their will and determination. Those who survive usually do so as stronger people. Not always better, but certainly stronger.

Betty admitted to feeling jealous of her brother's illness. "What I went through never showed. He stayed in the hospital and looked terribly sick and debilitated for a long time. He went bald and threw up after his chemotherapy and everyone made a big fuss over him.

"When I went through my depression, nothing showed on the outside, and I had the feeling that my parents and some of my friends were angry at me for 'feeling sorry for myself' when there was really nothing wrong with me. 'Just be glad you're not sick like Tommy,' they said— and of course, that made me madder and more depressed than ever.

"I came *very* close to suicide a few times. I had bought the pills and gone to the library and knew exactly how to do it. I finally got myself into therapy and was lucky enough to find a woman who was a good therapist as well as a kind human being. I felt as if she saved my life—in no less a way than the doctors at the hospital saved Tommy's life."

Betty is as much a survivor of a life-threatening illness as her brother. Therefore, she, more than his parents or any of his close friends, understands what he went through, and over the years they have developed an exceptionally close relationship.

Survivors of childhood cancer who say they feel different generally worry more about practical, reality-based things than they do about the fact that they might suffer a relapse or a second cancer. They are concerned about the genetic consequences of therapy, their reproductive capacities, their ability to maintain friendships with peers, changes that the cancer might necessitate in their academic and career choices, and the need for periodic medical monitoring.

The frequency and nature of posttreatment checkups vary, both with the length of time since the end of treatment and with the age of the child. Monthly trips to the outpatient clinic give way to semiannual ones and then to only once-a-year visits. Invasive procedures, such as spinal taps and bone marrow biopsies, are done less often, but when they are performed, they usually engender great anxiety. These procedures are, after all, the ones that diagnosed the disease in the first place, and they will thus forever be associated with devastating news. But as the years go by with no recurrence, survivors tend to think less and less about the experience.

One somewhat frightening aspect of survivorship is what psychologists call "adaptive denial," in which a survivor of cancer begins to feel almost invincible and starts taking foolish risks: smoking, engaging in unprotected sexual intercourse, playing dangerous sports—and missing appointments for checkups. When these kinds of "symptoms" appear, they should not be ignored. They are as indicative of a potentially serious problem as an abnormal blood test.

Survivors *do* think about the cancer reappearing. Many believe that a second bout of the disease would seriously erode the sense of hope that they have been able to maintain. Although the shock of having cancer might dissipate more quickly the second time around, the pain is no less acute than it was in the original disease. It may be even worse because with each new relapse, confidence in the hope of cure diminishes.

The second bout of cancer, whether it is a relapse of the original disease or an entirely new cancer, can be worse than the first. In fact, doctors are starting to see an increase in second cancers, probably because the survival rates from first cancers are now so good. This is truly an irony: a child survives cancer only to live with a higher-than-average risk of developing another type of cancer. Although no firm scientific data exist to prove or disprove this phenomenon, anecdotal evidence is strong.

True, there are fewer nasty surprises the second time around, but the feelings of bleakness and loneliness and sickness are perhaps even harder to bear when they are anticipated.

Survivors of childhood cancer are different from their peers who have not had the disease, and are more likely than those peers to seek psychological counseling. However, this finding should not be interpreted as a negative factor or as a precursor to emotional problems. Rather, it appears to represent an effort to deal positively and openly with stress and to learn from one's experiences. In fact, survivors talk about the positive consequences of having had cancer:

- An increased sense of mastery or confidence in one's ability to meet future challenges.
- A greater sensitivity to and empathy for the misfortunes and pain of others.
- A stronger sense of commitment to life's goals. Survivors of childhood cancer do not drop out of school, but neither do they continue activities that they see as useless or nonproductive. "Life is too short to do stupid things and to keep making the same mistakes over and over again," said one young man.
- A perceived need to contribute to the welfare of others. Many survivors choose health-related occupations and readily acknowledge that they do so out of a need to repay the "debt" of the kindness accorded them when they were ill.

Psychosocial Issues

Most survivors of childhood cancer lead lives that are the emotional envy of the rest of us. That is, they seem to have achieved a maturity far beyond their years.

Ian learned how to handle more than cancer. Or more to the point, he learned how to handle some of the changes that the cancer had wrought in his life. When he was in high school, he was attacked twice by what he called "gangs of black bully boys." The first time he felt helpless, because although he had begun to exercise and lift weights under his older brother's tutelage, he did not know how to fight. "I'd never been in a fight in my life, and when these guys jumped me, I was unprepared and didn't know what to do. So of course they creamed me, and I had to go to school the next day with two black eyes and a bunch of bruises."

Ian said that what was even worse than being beaten up for no reason by a bunch of strangers was feeling unable to do anything to protect himself. "I just sort of had to stand there and take it. Oh, I threw a few punches of my own, but I didn't know what I was doing."

He compared it to the experience of having had cancer as a little child. "This big, bad thing came out of nowhere and threatened my life, and the only thing I could do at the time was let them give me the treatment and try as hard as I could to get better."

Being assaulted on the steps of his high school simply because he is white felt to Ian like being attacked by cancer cells for an equally capricious reason. "That was when I decided to get into physical fitness in a big way," he said. "I started taking martial arts lessons. I learned to scuba dive, and I took wrestling lessons because my brothers always said that it was the hardest sport—in terms of the actual combat as well as the physical conditioning that you need to prepare for the matches."

Ian is something of a jock now. It's easy to see his strength, not because he looks muscle-bound, but because of the way he stands and the confidence he exudes. He is a gentle and mature young man of 20 years, and that, as much as his good physical condition, is what gives him strength.

The second time he was dragged into a fight was when he was a junior in high school, and this time he felt prepared. "I didn't want to get into it with these guys, but one of the girls from their gang starting hitting and slapping one of the girls I was with. It was at an after-hours event and the school guards had already left, so we were on our own.

"When the guys tried to break up the girls' fight, suddenly everyone was throwing punches. The police came eventually, and I was pretty beat up again, but this time I gave as good as I got, and I felt better about it."

Ian is not a person who goes looking for fights, but he is mature enough to realize that he lives in a world in which not everyone behaves the way he would like them to. "You have to be prepared for whatever bad stuff comes your way," he said. It was clear that he was talking about more than being attacked by gangs of young toughs.

As Ian is making an effort to grow into a strong, independent person, Sydney remains firmly attached to her parents. Although she no longer lives with them, she has been unable to separate what she wants and needs from what her parents want and need for her.

"My father wants me to go to graduate school and get a master's in computer science—and then go on for a doctorate," she said.

Why, when he knew what torture high school and college were for her because of her short-term memory loss?

"Because he wants me to be able to earn a living and have a good career, and you can make a lot of money in computers. He says it's where the future is."

Sydney's face was pinched with misery as she contemplated a great chunk of her life in graduate school. It was easy for a stranger to see her fear. Did her father not see it? Did he not care? And why, at age 26—a grown woman earning her own living, keeping her own house—did she not simply tell her father that she had no plans for graduate school?

"My father just doesn't understand," replied Sydney. "He didn't understand what I was going through when I was sick, and he doesn't understand now what it means to have had leukemia. Both he and my mother think that the whole thing is in the past and that I should just forget about it and get on with my life."

Sydney's family does not talk about feelings. "They're very uptight people," she explained. "They keep their upper lips stiff, and no one ever knows what's going on inside the family. Sometimes even the family doesn't know."

Sydney laughed wryly when she made the last statement, because her youngest brother, who is now in college, had not been born when she was being treated for leukemia. And because hers is a family that never discusses its experiences, that brother didn't know that anything out of the ordinary had happened to his big sister until she told him.

"I don't even know him," she said, referring to her younger brother. About her other brother, who is 3 years younger than Sydney, she said little. "We were never close. We never talked about the leukemia. We hardly talk now."

Many survivors are skittish about developing long-term relationships with other people, and some are rejected by potential spouses and/or lovers because of having had cancer. Beatrice talked about how jealous her boyfriend was of her relationship with the doctors and nurses at the clinic. "He thinks that I'm closer to them than I am to him. Maybe it's true." She paused to reflect for a moment. "But he hasn't gone through what they did with me. He never will."

Beatrice and her lover will need to talk about their feelings and the fact that providers of care to children with cancer perform services and develop relationships that even their parents do not and cannot share. It is a *different* relationship, not necessarily a better one.

Rose fell in love when she was 22 years old and just out of college. She and her young man dated for several months, and she felt that it was a solid, growing relationship. "But time went by and he wouldn't make a commitment," she said. "I asked him what was wrong: Didn't we like each other and have a good thing going and all that? 'Oh sure,' he said. He just didn't want to get serious, and he kept putting me off when I would try to talk about our relationship.

"Finally, one day, he just blurted out that he was afraid I was going to die."

Rose could not keep on with him after that, and now, 11 years later, she is strong and healthy, and he is married and a father. "Every once in a while, when I go down to North Carolina to visit my family, I see him at church, and it's obvious that he still feels something for me." She shrugs it off, but it's easy to see that the hurt is still there.

Although it may seem surprising, few survivors of childhood cancer say that their religious beliefs have undergone a significant change because of the illness. There are very few "seeing-a-sudden-light" conversions to a deeper faith, nor do many people lose faith in God because of being struck by a life-threatening illness. None of the literature on childhood cancer suggests a reason for this steadfastness of faith, but it is not difficult to ascribe it to the nature of faith itself. No explanation is needed or required.

However, if survivors feel as they always had about God, they feel very differently about themselves when the ordeal of acute illness and treatment is over. Most say they feel "special" in some way. Not better, just different. They feel that life has more meaning, greater clarity, and a preciousness that it did not have before the illness. They no longer take things for granted, and many of them feel as if they have a "debt" to pay to society for providing them the means to survive.

Employment Issues

Employment problems for survivors are widespread. Discrimination is common. In fact, in a National Cancer Institute survey of cancer survivors reported by Koocher and O'Malley (1981), 44% reported having been denied at least one job because of having had cancer in childhood. The American Cancer Society found that 90% of people who had cancer (not just children) experienced employment discrimination of some type.

Employers have serious concerns about survivors' eligibility for health insurance coverage. Small employers are particularly concerned because their premium rates are directly affected by the health problems of every single employee. Many companies will not hire a cancer survivor.

Even if the health insurance hurdle can be overcome, many employers fear that the survivor will have a high rate of absenteeism, will have a relapse, or will be too weak or too tired to do the job. None of these fears is valid.

Survivors also find that they are passed over for promotion (or even demoted), are not given raises at the same rate as other employees, and are the first to be laid off in the event of a reduction in force.

There are dozens of stated and tacit reasons for discriminating against survivors of child cancer. These reasons can all be fought legally, and there is a good chance of success. However, a legal battle of this nature can take years and is as depressing and exhausting as fighting the cancer itself. One woman said, "I took 3 sick days because I had the flu. It was the same flu that my officemate had and stayed out a week for. But I got fired. I decided to go through the federal Equal Employment Opportunity Commission instead of hiring a lawyer right away, and I ended up being angrier at the government bureaucrats than I was with the guy who fired me.

"The company ended up settling out of court, but the process took 2 years, and by that time I had another job. The hardest part was keeping my anger up for the whole time. It was so tempting to just forget it. But I'm stubborn and besides, I kind of felt that I owed it to other people in my situation.

"I didn't get a whole lot of money, but the guy who fired me was fired himself. That was the best part!"

It is against federal law to discriminate against employees who have had cancer *and* who have handicaps. The Americans With Disabilities Act is very specific about what an employer may and may not do with regard to the handicapped: He or she must meet the needs of disabled employees as long as those needs do not create "undue hardship" for the employer.

For example, the accommodations required of employers include making the workplace wheelchair accessible, permitting employees to work flexible schedules to allow for treatment-related absences, and letting employees work part-time or share jobs. Almost all survivors of childhood cancer are protected by the Americans With Disabilities Act even if they are not seriously physically disabled.

A less comprehensive but equally important law is the Federal Rehabilitation Act, which prohibits federal employers, or companies that receive any type of federal funding, from discriminating against handicapped workers, including cancer survivors. Many states also have laws that protect handicapped employees.

If you feel as if you have been discriminated against because you had cancer as a child, don't take it lying down! Anyone who has had the courage to fight a life-threatening disease has the courage to fight an unfair employer. In fact, one young man saw his lawsuit as part of the survival process.

"I was smarter than practically everybody else in my office, I was in physically better shape because I go to the gym three times a week, and I was good at my job."

But when Jim's boss found out that he had Hodgkin's disease (the insurance company refused to add him to the group policy), he was fired. "'Good-bye and good luck,' was what he basically said," Jim reported. "He wasn't even particularly nice about it.

"Luckily, I knew what my rights were because a girl I had gone through treatment with was having trouble getting a job and she told me who to contact. When my ex-boss found out that I was filing charges, he called me up at home and apologized and offered me my job back."

Even though he has no respect for the man who fired him in the first place, Jim went back to work because he needed the money and "I wanted to prove to this guy that those of us who have survived cancer are just as good as anyone else."

Health Insurance

Most childhood cancer survivors were covered on their parents' health insurance policies when they fell ill. Eventually, though, when they are no longer their parents' dependents, they will be dropped from the policy and will have to find their own insurance coverage.

Purchasing health insurance is not impossible, especially if the policy is issued through the survivor's employer. The preexisting condition clause will apply to all claims arising from the cancer for a certain period of time, usually the first 1 to 3 years after the coverage takes effect. This means that the carrier will not pay such claims for that period of time, and most carriers will require medical certification that the cancer is cured or at least in long-term remission.

It is unlikely that anyone who is actively suffering from cancer at the time he or she makes application for health insurance will be given a policy.

Health insurance should be a primary consideration when looking for a job or thinking about changing jobs. In fact, it is unwise to leave a job where you have good coverage for one that either does not offer health insurance as an employee benefit (40 million Americans are in this position) or offers insurance benefits that are significantly less comprehensive than those you already have.

Do not be shy about discussing health insurance during a job interview. Everyone else does. Pat said she made a big mistake when she was looking for her first job after college. "The man who was going to be my boss knew that I'd had leukemia—because I told him. But after that, I didn't want to mention it again because I didn't want him to think that was all I thought about, or that I walked around all day waiting to get sick again.

"So I never asked anything about the health insurance—and the company never gave me any. It never occurred to me at the time that I was being discriminated against, but it was a small outfit, and they just never signed me up. Their insurer didn't know I existed. I was too naive to realize that there were forms to fill out. My parents had always taken care of that stuff when I had leukemia.

"When I got my foot caught in a bus door and broke my toe, I went to the emergency room and of course, the first thing they asked for was my insurance information. I gave them the Blue Cross card that I'd had for ages, but it was from years before when I was covered by my parents.

"Right there in the emergency room, I found out that I had absolutely no health insurance *at all!*"

Pat forced her employer to put her on the company's policy, but they didn't want to because she had had cancer. Her boyfriend talked her into threatening to sue, which she did. "I hated getting into that kind of a relationship with them, but I was mad." The company acquiesced because they knew they would lose a legal fight, but they fired Pat shortly thereafter on trumped-up charges of incompetence. Again, her boyfriend encouraged her to sue. "I just couldn't. I don't have the energy for that kind of stuff anymore. Besides, I had found another job. But you can bet your bottom dollar that I know exactly what my health benefits are now!"

When you receive health insurance coverage, you will be given a copy of the policy. Read it. Even the fine print. It will explain what the policy will and will not pay for, and it can be used as a source of "proof" if you have a disagreement with the carrier about the terms of coverage. The policy is a legal contract, and you can hold the company to its terms if a justified claim is denied.

Individual health insurance is much harder to obtain than a group policy. In fact, fewer and fewer companies offer individual policies, and most of those that do will refuse to insure someone with a major preexisting condition.

Physical Effects

The price of long-term survival and cure for some children is that the treatment that saved their lives can have some less-than-pleasant consequences. These consequences can be devastating because they represent yet another physical and emotional hurdle, probably a permanent one.

Late or long-term effects depend on the type of cancer and the nature of the treatment.

Growth and Development

Many children suffer from diminution of linear growth (the length of limbs or overall height), which is usually permanent and may even be progressive. Although the presence and extent of growth retardation vary widely, this effect is especially common after a child under the age of 5 has been treated with cranial radiation.

Children who have had radiation for localized tumors may experience limb shortening or distortion of the vertebrae due to damaged muscles that pull the spinal column out of alignment.

Both Kate and Alan are short. Kate is 5 feet tall and Alan is 5 feet, 3 inches. However, the difference in their sexes makes a huge difference in the way they react to their stature.

Kate is only a little shorter than average for a young woman. She might have been short anyway, even without the radiation (she was adopted when she was an infant so she doesn't know the height range of her biological family). She doesn't appear little when one first meets her, perhaps because she is not a "small" person. Her intelligence, maturity, and sensitivity are such that one soon forgets that she has a physical "disability." In all other respects, except for her deformed eye, Kate is physically ordinary.

Alan, on the other hand, is not only short, he looks at least 6 or

7 years younger than his 20 years. He has no beard, his face has not lost the "puppylike" characteristics of prepuberty, and his voice has not changed.

This could be a disaster for a young man just finishing his sophomore year in college. Alan is uncomfortable talking about his feelings, so it is hard to know how much his physical appearance affects his life. It must be considerable. He is outwardly a cheerful person, almost evangelical in his insistence that he is not afraid of the future and not hampered by the past, but it is not difficult to believe, in this instance at least, that Alan is a depressed and unhappy young man behind the facade.

Osteoporosis is also a long-term effect. This condition, usually seen in older people (most commonly, postmenopausal women), results in decreased bone density, making bones lighter and more porous, and thus subject to a higher risk of fracture.

Reproduction

To some, it may seem ironic that a person who has survived cancer in childhood would want to have children of his or her own. If one's own early years were filled with pain, fear, and desperate illness, why risk inflicting the same fate on one's own children? Most cancer survivors don't see it this way at all. What they worry about is *not* being able to have children or, if they can, about passing on a genetic defect as a result of the chemotherapy and/or radiation.

These are reasonable and rational questions, but not enough research has been conducted to provide definitive answers to them. However, because the chemotherapeutic agents used to treat cancer interfere with cellular metabolism and cell division, there is reason to suspect that they *might* cause mutation or some other kind of genetic damage, all of which, it is safe to assume, is dose dependent.

Although it is known that anticancer drugs cause genetic damage to some human cells, it is not known whether these drugs damage germ cells (the ones responsible for reproduction). Little research has been done on the sensitivity of human gonads to mutagens (agents such as drugs that can be responsible for genetic mutations). For obvious reasons, such studies cannot be undertaken with human subjects, and it seems clear that laboratory animals do not respond to exposure to mutagenics in the same way that humans do. Thus, the question of whether cancer treatment impairs human reproduction remains unanswered.

There has, however, been some anecdotal evidence of germ cell depletion in men, as well as abnormal endocrine function as a result of radiation and chemotherapy. Although it is unusual for adolescent boys to think far enough into the future to be concerned about fatherhood, it is possible to collect and freeze sperm before treatment begins. Patients should be told about sperm banking and offered this option.

Victor thinks he might be sterile, but he has no plans to find out until he meets, falls in love with, and proposes to a woman. "If I have my sperm count tested now, when there's no practical reason to know, then I might have to give up hope of ever having children."

The effect of chemotherapy and radiation in women is harder to determine because ovarian function is more complicated to test than sperm production. However, whatever the effects, it is certain that they are dose dependent and probably irreversible. Other late effects in women include a decreased libido, amenorrhea and other symptoms of menopause, and diminished breast development.

The effect of radiation and chemotherapy on fertility is almost impossible to evaluate because adolescents undergoing treatment usually do not become pregnant, and if they do, abortion is common. Pregnancy after treatment has been discontinued is an "iffy" area. Fetuses that have been aborted are not usually tested for abnormal cell development, and there have been no definitive studies of children born of survivors of childhood cancer because there have been too few long-term survivors. This situation will change in the future.

From anecdotal evidence, however, it seems reasonable to say that there is a real risk of congenital abnormalities for the offspring of childhood cancer survivors.

The only real data that exist are severely limited because the conditions considered bear little resemblance to what happens to children with cancer. For example, observers have found no statistically significant effects of parental exposure to ionizing radiation on the children of Japanese survivors of atomic bomb blasts at Hiroshima and Nagasaki.

The offspring of the Japanese survivors were examined for a variety of factors that might indicate genetic damage (congenital malformation, stillbirth, chromosomal rearrangement, gender ratio). No results could be attributed to the parents' exposure to radiation.

There are drawbacks that prevent our drawing a sigh of relief over these findings, however. In the first place, the Japanese survivors were exposed to radiation only, not to drug therapy. The amount of exposure varied enormously, depending on their distance from the blasts. Moreover, the conditions under which the retrospective studies were done were certainly not ideal in terms of eliminating other factors that might have had a bearing on the outcome.

Kate has a 2-year-old boy and is pregnant. "I always knew I would be able to have children," she said, "because my periods were regular and I've never had any problem with them.

"But I was told to have all the children I wanted before I turn 30 because there has been some research about the late effects of the chemotherapy I had. I was told that I probably would have a very early menopause. But who knows," she added with a shrug. "Between now and then, research can show a million different things. You know how doctors are always changing their minds."

Kate said that she always wanted to be a mother. "That's the career I had chosen for myself. I never wanted to do anything else."

But what if she had been sterile?

"I would have adopted," she said.

Cognitive Functioning

Radiation to the head and spinal cord, as well as some chemotherapeutic agents, can affect cognitive and sensory abilities in addition to both long- and short-term memory. This means that the child may not appear to be as smart as he or she was before the treatment and may have problems with hearing, vision, and other sensory functions. One of the more distressing aspects of these changes is that they often do not become apparent until 3 or more years after treatment.

The more immature the developing brain at the time of treatment, the more likely the appearance of cognitive problems after treatment. It is impossible, however, to predict the exact nature and extent of the retardation, because so much depends on the type of medication and the dose, as well as on individual factors that are as yet not understood.

Many affected children have difficulty paying attention and learning to read and do mathematics, skills that depend heavily on memory. It is not uncommon for IQ scores to drop as much as 20 points, especially when the child received cranial radiation before the age of 5. The amount of radiation exposure also affects the type and extent of cognitive dysfunction. Some trouble signs include the following:

- Declining grades in some or all school subjects
- Decreased legibility of handwriting
- Diminished reading or math skills
- Hearing or vision problems
- Difficulty with written language
- Decreased attention span

Although there is no reason why children with memory loss and lowered IQ cannot continue to learn, they will do so at a slower rate. Parents must once again serve as advocates to see that their child receives an adequate education.

Alan has a problem with short-term memory, but both in high school and now in college, he has been lucky enough to participate in a remedial studies program. "The people who run the program have taught me all kinds of tricks and techniques to remember things. Before they began to help me, I would read my texts for school and I'd be pretty sure I knew all the material. But the next day, the day of the test, when I woke up in the morning, everything would be gone!"

Kate said she can't do math. "But lots of people can't," she said with a laugh. "Besides, when you're an adult and out of school, what do you need math for?"

Sydney also has problems with both math and short-term memory. She, however, has not been able to manage the aftereffects as well as some of the other survivors interviewed. She works for a computer software company and writes programs for elementary education. She acknowledges that hers is probably not the best choice of careers. "I have a hard time communicating with people—that is, telling them what a program means or what it can do for them. It's not doing the work that bothers me, it's talking about it and explaining it."

Sydney has trouble remembering details, which in itself causes problems for her in such a detail-oriented industry, but she has not yet come to grips with the fact that she must either find a way around her shortcomings or find another career.

For instance, she almost missed a business appointment. She was to meet someone for lunch at noon at a restaurant only a few steps from her office. "The guy called and asked if I had forgotten. I hadn't, but I don't have a clock in my office, and I was so absorbed in my work that I didn't realize that the morning had gone by. I rushed out and met him and it was okay."

If there is no clock in her office, why doesn't she use the one built into her computer—or wear a watch?

Sydney seemed nonplussed when that suggestion was made—as if the thought had not occurred to her. She shrugged and looked sheepish, and one had the feeling that she would not wear a watch, she would keep on missing appointments—and would eventually lose this job, as she has lost two previous ones because of problems like these.

Physical Deformities

Koocher and O'Malley (1981) report that women with physical handicaps as a result of childhood cancer (and for other reasons as well) are less likely to marry than women without such long-term physical effects. With men, it is the opposite. Those with handicaps are more likely to marry than nonimpaired men.

This probably has more to do with societal expectations and cultural norms than with the fact of having had cancer. Society expects women to look a certain way, and if they do not, they are seen as less than desirable. Men are expected to achieve a certain look also, but if they do not, they are "allowed" to develop other assets that replace physical perfection.

The only solution to this unjust situation, it seems, is for female cancer survivors with physical deformities to behave the way other physically "undesirable" women (those who are too fat, too thin, too plain, too awkward, and so forth) have for ages—develop their inner selves and go about their lives as if the physical scars and imperfections don't matter. Because they don't.

Kate has a seriously deformed eye. When she was 3 years old, she was diagnosed with rhabdomyosarcoma in the muscle of her right eye. It was treated with heavy doses of both radiation and chemotherapy, which destroyed the optic nerve on that side and stopped the growth of both the bony orbit and the eyelid. Years later, she received a false eye that was fitted over the sightless eye in order to avoid removing the eye.

She wears her shoulder-length brown hair in a swoop that covers her eye and shields it somewhat. If she can, Kate positions herself so that her "good" side faces the person she is with.

She said that dealing with the deformity was much harder when she was younger. "You know how cruel some kids can be," she said. Some schoolmates made fun of her, but most accepted her as she was and quickly ignored the eye. Strangers were worse. "They would come up to me and say things like, 'What's the matter little girl, did you poke a stick in your eye?' "

Now that she is an adult, do people stare and ask what happened? "No, they ask [my husband] Mark."

Kate is relieved that she doesn't have to bear the entire burden of explanation, and sometimes she is amused that whereas people are afraid to mention it to her, they have no qualms about asking her husband. "If they think they might hurt my feelings, why don't they just ignore it altogether?"

Joan's hair didn't grow back completely after cranial radiation. She has been in remission for 9 years, but until 4 years ago, she continued to wear a wig. Her hair loss is quite noticeable, but she is so pretty that one forgets about it almost immediately. She stopped wearing a wig only because her family encouraged her to. "They told me I look fine, and now I'm starting to experiment with different ways to wear my hair so that it looks fuller."

About 15 years or so after Victor completed treatment, he began having fainting episodes that were preceded by a period of wild tachycardia, during which his heart rate would suddenly jump to 180 or 190. This happened several times and was completely unpredictable.

Finally, he was put on medication to which he reacted unfavorably. "My heart just started deteriorating," he said. "I couldn't work, I could hardly breathe, and I couldn't sleep unless I was propped up on four or five pillows."

So badly had Victor's heart deteriorated that he was hospitalized and became a candidate for a heart transplant. During that time, he was taken off all medication and the condition of his heart improved and strengthened to the point that he did not need a transplant.

But he still had episodes of severe tachycardia and fainting, which were treated by an automatic internal defibrillator, a device that senses when his heart is about to race itself into a dangerous state. The defibrillator, which lies just under Victor's skin and is attached to his heart muscle by tiny wires, shocks the heart in the same way a doctor does externally. (In television movies, the doctor applies paddles to a patient's chest, yells "Stand clear!" and a jolt of electricity restarts the heart.)

When Victor recovered sufficiently to return to the cancer center in New York where he had originally been treated and where he goes for an annual checkup, he told his oncologist about his cardiac problems. "Oh, yes," she said to Victor. "We've had several cases of sudden, unexplained death as a result of one of the chemotherapy drugs you were taking."

She told Victor that he was lucky to be alive.

Relapse

If the cancer reappears, everyone is devastated. Fantasies of a cure become harder to maintain and hope diminishes. Often, everyone feels like a failure—just as they were starting to feel like a success and life was returning to normal. "It felt like the beginning of the end," said one adolescent. "I really thought that this time I was going to die." She did not.

Anger and guilt run rampant. Parents feel guilty because they fear that they didn't take good enough care of their child, siblings remember all the mean thoughts they had about the sick child during the illness, the child feels that perhaps he or she didn't try hard enough to get better or didn't have a sufficiently positive attitude. And everyone is angry at the doctors and nurses for not curing the disease.

God also gets a healthy share of these negative feelings.

When relapse occurs, maintenance treatment is stopped and induction treatment is reinstituted. The medications and doses may be different from those used the first time, but their goal is the same: to kill the cancer cells and shrink the tumor. Although the likelihood of good response to treatment decreases the second time around, the chances of remission are still excellent.

A separate but related problem is the phenomenon of second (different) cancers. Although very few long-term studies have been conducted because long-term cancer survival is such a recent phenomenon, doctors believe that survivors of childhood cancer are between 10 and 20 times more likely to get cancer as adults than are people who did not have the disease as a child. Although the incidence of second cancer depends on the type of the first cancer, it is believed that survivors of Hodgkin's disease are especially at risk.

Again, no one knows why this is so, but it seems reasonable to assume that all the risk factors that existed at the time of the first cancer, plus the risk factors involved in the treatment, may have a cumulative effect, thereby increasing the overall risk of a second cancer.

Rehabilitation

Rehabilitation is the effort to restore, maintain, or prevent further decline in body function. The process begins with a series of assessment tests to determine the amount of function lost and the likelihood of either restoring it or retraining other nerves and muscles to perform the lost functions.

The amount of rehabilitation necessary, and its ultimate success, depend to a great extent on the age of the child at diagnosis and treatment. The younger the child, the greater the degree of growth and development retardation, *but* the more pliant the child and the easier to retrain.

In addition to various exercises and physical therapy regimens, rehabilitation consists of learning to adapt to braces, crutches, and prostheses. Rehabilitation should be initiated at the same time treatment is begun in order to combat fatigue, weakness, and pain.

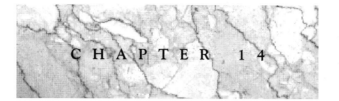

Ethical Issues

Ethical issues arise from conflicts about making moral decisions. When treatment for childhood cancer is at the foundation of the issues, the decisions will have long-lasting, if not permanent, effects. Such decisions involve the need to discriminate, not between right and wrong, but between two positive or beneficial courses of action.

It is easy to say, and to believe, that parents always want to do the right thing for their children. This statement has two immediate and obvious problems. First, it is not always true. Stories of deliberate and inadvertent child abuse and neglect are so common that people have become almost inured to them. We will not deal with out-and-out wrongdoing here, not because we want to sweep it under the rug, but because we make the assumption that the readers of this book do not fall into that class of people.

The second problem is that although parents may *want* to do right, the correct course of action is not always clear. For example, which would be in the child's best interest: to amputate a leg to ensure that the entire tumor has been removed, or to salvage the limb but run the risk of a relapse or metastasis? As another example, what if an adolescent and his or her parents are in conflict over treatment? Can and should the parents force a course of action against the child's will?

Some of these issues and questions will be explored herein, but we will not—cannot—tell you what to do.

First, who is a child?

Simple, you say. He or she is the product of my body (or the "gift" of someone else via the adoption process), a young person for whom I am responsible.

This is true in an emotional sense, but in a medical-legal sense, the issue is more complex.

Legally, a child is anyone under 18 years old. This means that a child cannot sign a contract, is not liable for incurred financial debts, and cannot give permission to receive medical treatment. A person under 18 who lacks parents or a legal guardian "belongs" to the state.

However, children of any age are not chattel, and pediatric oncologists do not treat them as if they were. In fact, these physicians are coming to believe that children of almost any age—except perhaps those younger than 6 or 7 years of age—should participate in decisions about their treatment. If procedures are explained carefully, most children can understand them and give their assent, which, however, is not the same as legal consent for treatment.

Moreover, children around 14 years of age and older can and do give consent for treatment independent of their parents. It is not technically legal, but most pediatric oncology centers treat older children as if they were adults when it comes to including them in the decision-making process. They are considered "mature minors."

An "emancipated minor," on the other hand, is a person who, while still under age 18, meets certain other criteria and is therefore considered legally a full adult. Those criteria include marriage, parenthood, service in the armed forces, or the condition of being self-supporting and living apart from one's parents.

Making Decisions

Some decisions do not matter at all (what to eat in a restaurant), some matter very much but are neither permanent nor devastating if wrong (choosing a college, buying one stock rather than another, taking a job), and others are a matter of life and death—quite literally, in the case of making treatment decisions.

Five moral principles can be used when making an important decision: respect for persons, beneficence, nonmaleficence, proportionality, and justice.

Respect for persons implies that everyone has the right to autonomy and self-determination. In the case of young children, this right is not abrogated; rather, it is vested in the parents. That is, parents must make decisions based on what the child would want if he or she *could* make the decision autonomously. Respect for persons implies that we are obligated to protect those with diminished autonomy: the mentally retarded, the old and senile—and children.

Beneficence is the obligation to take positive steps to do good—to provide the treatment that will result in the greatest chance for cure. *Nonmaleficence* is the duty to do as little harm as possible. *Proportionality* implies the need to balance benefits and risks in order to decrease harm and enhance good. This is often easier said than done.

Justice is the attempt to distribute society's benefits and burdens fairly, which does not necessarily mean equally. Although equals should be treated equally, it is the responsibility of the person or agency distributing the burdens and benefits to justify differences in the way people are treated. For example, why is Johnny receiving this or that treatment when Jackie, who has the same disease, is not?

When Parents Refuse Treatment for Children

Although courts in the United States are by no means consistent, when parents refuse traditional medical care for their children, the general trend is to determine the best course of action to protect the child—that is, to create an end result that will provide the most comfort and the best quality of life regardless of whether a cure is possible.

This works the other way too. Sometimes, when every known treatment has been tried and has failed, and when nothing further can be done for the child, some parents want doctors to keep on trying: to attempt more and more drastic procedures that will produce nothing but pain and discomfort for the child. Under such circumstances, doctors and hospitals have been known to go to court to stop treatment. The justification is that in the terminal phase of illness, rest and comfort—rather than further attempts at treatment—are in the best interest of the child.

When parents refuse traditional treatment, courts usually try to examine the main issue: whether the child will be deprived of life-sustaining benefits. In other words, a judge will want to know the "track record" of the treatment under consideration. If the treatment is too new to be evaluated, or if it has been only marginally successful in the past, courts are not likely to force parents to consent to it. But if the treatment is known to be successful and the parents refuse it for a variety of "irrational" reasons, the court will probably order them to consent. In fact, there is now enough legal precedent to make that decision a foregone conclusion. Parents may not deny their children a reasonable try for life.

When adolescents refuse treatments that their parents want them to have, the conflict is not only between patient and health care provider, but also between parent and child. Age makes a significant difference in the way such a conflict is resolved. If an adolescent demonstrates sound understanding of what the consequences of refusal are, if he or she is mature enough and has thought the problem through thoroughly, then his or her desire should be taken seriously.

In these cases, it is important for the patient, the physicians, and the parents to sit down and discuss things fully and openly and for everyone to *listen* to one another's point of view. Usually the problem can be resolved in this manner. Sometimes an outside arbitrator can be brought in—and rarely does the case go to court.

Confidentiality

It should go without saying that all patients' medical records, and all information revealed to health care professionals by patients, should be kept confidential. When the patient is a child, however, confidentiality is sometimes seen as less important than when the patient is an adult. This is clearly wrong. It flies in the face of respect for the child as a person.

Legal status as a minor does not negate the duty of health professionals to protect the confidentiality of patients. When a patient gives information to a doctor that is unknown to the patient's parents (about drug or alcohol use, sexual activity, and the like), there is no reason for the doctor to tell the parents.

Protection of confidentiality can be difficult in a large teaching hospital, where so many people have access to patients' charts. However, if parents or patients become aware of deliberate or inadvertent leaks of information, they should make certain that the hospital is made aware of what is happening. For example, employees who discuss patients in the elevator or in the cafeteria should be cautioned of the inappropriateness of such behavior. In some instances, serious breaches of confidentiality can be grounds for dismissal of an employee or even legal action.

Participation in Medical Research

Medical research on humans, also known as clinical trials, consists of an experiment, or a series of experiments, designed to answer a medical question. Such experiments, also known as *protocols*, use established scientific methods to test a hypothesis: for instance, is a new drug better than an existing one to treat a certain disease? Or, if a new drug is as good as existing ones, does it work with fewer side effects?

There are two major types of medical research: therapeutic and nontherapeutic. The former provides direct benefit to the subject, whereas the latter provides only general information and might possibly help others. We are concerned here with therapeutic research.

Clinical trials are divided into three phases. *Phase I* is designed to test the toxicity of an experimental agent and to determine the maximum tolerated dose. This phase represents the first time a drug has been used on human beings. Children are almost never used in Phase I trials.

Phase II tests the activity of the experimental agent against the type of disease for which it is intended. In terms of children with cancer, there has lately been a move to rely on drugs still in Phase II trials when all else has failed, or to use them to manage patients in the terminal phase of an illness. Researchers sometimes urge participation in Phase II trials as a "last ditch" effort. "It's this or nothing," parents sometimes are told, and researchers have been known to present participation in the research as if there were no choice.

Phase III trials compare one treatment with another—or with no treatment. This phase is almost always conducted as double-blind research—that is, neither the researcher nor the patient knows which subjects are receiving the agent under study.

In the course of her work as a medical writer, Sarah came to know a number of biochemists and other researchers. She respected them and their work. But the day she found out that her son Les had acute lymphoblastic leukemia (ALL), she was exposed to a different side of the way they function.

"That first morning, when Les was in a hospital way on the other side of the country and I was here in Philadelphia trying to make these decisions on which his *life* depended, I got a call from a man at NIH. He said he had been called by a colleague of his whom I had called to ask for advice about Les.

"This guy said he'd heard that my son had just been diagnosed and he wanted him for one of his leukemia protocols. He also said that I should call the doctors at the hospital in Portland, where they were trying to stabilize Les so we could fly him home, and tell them not to give Les any cancer drugs because then he would be ineligible for his protocol.

"Can you imagine the nerve—the insensitivity! On my son's first day after diagnosis, when I hadn't even begun to try to assimilate what had happened to us, here was this guy calling up with a recruitment speech. I don't know how I managed to keep my temper, but I told him that I wasn't at all sure that I wanted my son to participate in medical research and that I'd have to get back to him.

"I never did, and I never heard from him again."

Sarah was outraged, not because of the need to have her son participate in a research protocol, but because of the way he was recruited. "It reminded me of that old World War II poster of Uncle Sam, with his face all grim, pointing his finger and making you feel guilty if you didn't join the Army that minute."

What happened to Sarah is probably not an isolated or unusual event. Medical research, with its attendant competition for grant money, academic publication, and collegial recognition, is an almost dog-eat-dog endeavor. As in all such efforts, sometimes the "consumer" is treated shabbily. Although researchers have their subjects' best interests at heart, their zeal to do science can sometimes overshadow their acknowledgment of those subjects as human beings—especially vulnerable ones, in the case of childhood cancer. Again, it is ultimately up to parents to guard their child's safety and welfare.

However, with almost no exceptions, all the standard treatments in use today that so dramatically save the lives of children with cancer are available because they were tested and proved effective in clinical trials.

If your child is asked to participate in research, you will be given a copy of the protocol, which is a written guideline that describes how the experiment is to be conducted. You and your child will read—in understandable language, not "medicalese"—what the objectives are, who is eligible to participate, how the study is designed, what will happen, and when and what the entire plan of the experiment is. You will also be told something about the results of animal and early human studies, what side effects to expect, and what the toxic effects might be.

You, as well as the child if he or she is old enough, will then be asked to sign a formal written consent. This is a serious decision and should not be undertaken lightly.

Why should you offer your child as a research subject? There are a number of reasons. Children and adolescents need to participate in cancer research because in many respects, young people are physiologically different from adults.

On the other hand, ethical principles preclude forcing individuals to serve as research subjects against their will. This creates a conflict. Ethical considerations, psychological and emotional competence to consent, the possibility of harm, and parental and societal attitudes must all be evaluated.

Although it may be fairly easy to agree in principle that medical research is a good thing (after all, the ever-improving survival rates of childhood cancer would not have been possible without such research), one's own child is neither a principle nor an abstract idea.

The National Commission for the Protection of Human Subjects of Biomedical and Behavioral Research (henceforth called the National Commission) has established guidelines about who can give consent to participate in research. Every institution that receives federal funds (almost every hospital in the country falls into this category) must comply with these guidelines. In the case of children, the National Commission has established standards regarding their ability to understand the risks and benefits of participation in research, thus enabling them to give informed consent.

Those standards include the child's cognitive development, a comparison of the ability of children and adolescents with that of adults to understand the ramifications of participation, and the child's level of moral reasoning and the factors that influence it.

It almost goes without saying that participation in medical research must be completely voluntary, and children must be allowed to veto their parents' decision to "volunteer" them as subjects. In fact, the National Commission makes a major point of this: a child's veto should be binding unless there is absolutely no other choice and his or her life will be placed in serious jeopardy unless he or she is given the experimental agent.

Researchers and physicians have expressed a wide range of opinions about the issue of children assenting to or vetoing participation. Parents also disagree with one another and with their physicians about this issue. The role of parents in encouraging or discouraging their children's participation in research depends to a large extent on parents' moral values and psychological makeup, and on the way the research project is presented to them, which in turn depends on the values and psychology of the researcher.

Consent may be withdrawn *any* time after it has been given—even after the research has begun.

Resources

The resources in this appendix are not intended to be a complete list of everything that is available and understandable in "ordinary" language. Rather, the items listed here are a starting point for readers interested in knowing more.

Every organization and agency has personnel who will be more than glad to provide additional information. Other sources include public libraries, hospital libraries (although they tend to have highly technical references), college and university libraries, and organizations that are not widely known outside local areas.

General Information on Childhood Cancer

ᴥ The National Cancer Institute (NCI; Building 31, National Institutes of Health, Bethesda, Maryland 20892) maintains the Cancer Information Service network, which provides up-to-date information. Trained professional and volunteer staff operate this toll-free telephone service (800-4-CANCER [800-422-6237]) to answer questions about the causes and nature of cancer. NCI also has a wide variety of free publications, as well as information about medical facilities, physician referral suggestions, and other cancer-related resources.

- The National Health Information Center (800-336-4797) has a list of more than 1,100 health organizations related to an almost unlimited number of diseases, including childhood cancer.
- For a list of national public and private health service organizations, contact Resource Information Guide, P.O. Box 990297, Redding, California 96099.
- The National Self-Help Clearinghouse will give you support group information if you send a stamped, self-addressed envelope to 25 West 43rd Street, New York, New York 10036.
- Physician Data Query (PDQ) is a computerized information service that gives both doctors and patients access to the latest cancer treatment information from both U.S. and international cancer treatment centers. PDQ includes information about the staging system, treatment options, and prognosis for long-term survival. It also has information on where clinical trials are being administered and which physicians in the caller's area offer the latest treatments. Call 800-4-CANCER (800-422-6237) and request a free PDQ search for cancer treatment information.
- The National Bone Marrow Donor Registry, administered by the American Red Cross in association with the American Association of Blood Banks and the Council of Community Blood Centers, maintains a computerized list of bone marrow donors identified by tissue type.
- The Cetus Oncology Resource Guide is available in many public and hospital libraries. This guide contains information about organizations concerned with cancer; it includes a section on childhood cancer.

If you have a computer with a modem, you can access several health databases, some of which are easily comprehensible by the average layperson.

- Grateful Med, a database at the National Library of Medicine, is a compilation of 3,600 medical journals for in-depth searches on any medical subject. Call 800-638-8480 to order the software or 301-496-6308 for a free demonstration disk and brochure.

- The *Directory of Online Healthcare Databases* is available by calling 503-471-1627.
- The Health Reference Center is a commercial database of 4,000 consumer and medical publications. For the branch nearest you, call 800-227-8431.
- For a list of health-oriented computer bulletin boards, contact Black Bag BBS, 1 Ball Farm Way, Wilmington, Delaware 19808. With a modem, call 302-994-3772.

Voluntary Organizations

- Candlelighters Childhood Cancer Foundation
  7910 Woodmont Avenue, Suite 460
  Bethesda, Maryland 20814
  301-657-8401
- American Cancer Society (national headquarters)
  19 West 56th Street
  New York, New York 10019
  212-586-8700
- Leukemia Society of America (national headquarters)
  733 Third Avenue
  New York, New York 10017
  212-573-8484
- Corporate Angel Network (free air transport to medical care)
  Westchester County Airport, Building One
  White Plains, New York 10604
  914-328-1313
- Ronald McDonald House (national headquarters)
  Golin-Harris Communications, Inc.
  500 North Michigan Avenue
  Chicago, Illinois 60611
  312-836-7114
- Make-A-Wish Foundation of America
  2600 North Central Avenue, Suite 936

Phoenix, Arizona 85004
602-240-6600
❧ Association for Research of Childhood Cancer
P.O. Box 251
Buffalo, New York 14225-0251
716-681-4433
❧ Hole in the Wall Gang Camp
565 Ashford Canter Road
P.O. Box 98
Ashford, Connecticut 06278
203-429-3444
❧ Camp Simcha (for Orthodox Jewish children primarily, but not exclusively)
48 West 25th Street
New York, New York 10010
212-255-1160
❧ Special Love, Inc. (Camp Fantastic)
117 Youth Development Court
Winchester, Virginia 22602
703-667-3774
❧ National Coalition of Cancer Survivorship
1010 Wayne Avenue
Silver Spring, Maryland 20910
301-650-8868

Employment Issues

❧ American Cancer Society (has state-specific information about employment discrimination)
❧ National Coalition for Cancer Survivorship (provides a limited attorney referral service)
❧ Your state legislator, congressional representative, or senator
❧ League of Women Voters
❧ Equal Employment Opportunity Commission (has regional offices around the country)

- President's Committee on the Employment of People With Disabilities (800-526-7234)
- U.S. Department of Health and Human Services, Office for Civil Rights
- U.S. Department of Labor, Office of Federal Contract Compliance Programs (has regional offices)
- U.S. Department of Labor, Office of Pension and Welfare Benefits (regarding discrimination by an employer or union)

Organizations That Recommend Specialists for a Second Medical Opinion

- Cancer Information Service of the National Cancer Institute (800-4-CANCER [800-422-6237])
- American Cancer Society (local offices)
- Community Clinical Oncology Programs (CCOPS; supported by the National Cancer Institute)
- Regional cancer centers designated by the National Cancer Institute
- American College of Surgeons
- Second opinion centers established by all major private insurance companies

Insurance Issues

The National Consumer Insurance Organization (121 North Payne Street, Alexandria, Virginia 22314) publishes a number of helpful brochures about insurance issues. Other publications that might prove useful include the following:

- "Comprehensive Health Insurance for High-Risk Individuals," available from

Cancer Support Services
2626 East 82nd Street, Suite 325
Minneapolis, Minnesota 55425

➤ "The Consumer's Guide to Disability Insurance" and "The Consumer's Guide to Health Insurance," both available from

Health Insurance Association of America
1025 Connecticut Avenue, N.W.
Washington, DC 20036

➤ "Health Insurance: Risk Pools" (Publication number HRD-88-66BR), available from

U.S. General Accounting Office
P.O. Box G015
Gaithersburg, Maryland 20877

Glossary

Alternative medical treatment   Remedies that fall outside the mainstream of the health care system; usually have not been tested by accepted scientific protocols that ensure safety and efficacy

Amputation   Removal of a body part, usually referring to limbs

Anorexia   Loss of appetite

Antibody   A molecule of protein manufactured by the body as a reaction to an antigen

Antigen   A foreign (to a particular body) protein substance

Anxiety   Distress or uneasiness of mind caused by apprehension and/or fear; a state of psychic tension in the face of real or imagined danger

Art therapy   The process of interpreting and analyzing feelings and emotions expressed by drawing, sketching, painting, sculpting, and other art forms

Aspiration   Insertion of a needle into tissue to draw out cells for microscopic study

Assent   Giving "passive" permission for a medical procedure by not objecting to it

Autonomic nervous system   The system containing nerves that regulate involuntary body processes such as respiration and digestion

Benign   Not malignant

Biopsy   Microscopic examination of cells to determine the presence of cancer

Bone marrow   Soft tissue in the hollow of long bones where red blood cells and other types of cells are produced

Carcinogen   A substance that causes cancer

Carcinogenesis   The cause and origin of cancer

Case manager   A person, often a nurse, employed by an insurance company or an HMO, who follows patients with expensive and/or long-term health problems; the goal is to find the best care at the least expensive cost

CT (computed tomography) scan   A diagnostic X-ray technique in which minor differences in the body's absorption of X rays can be enhanced by computer to create a picture of both soft and hard tissues; sometimes called a CAT (computed axial tomography) scan

Catheter   A plastic tube of varying lengths that leads from inside the body (the bladder, a blood vessel) to the outside; used either to drain body fluids or to introduce a fluid into the body

Cell   A mass of protoplasm that contains a nucleus; the basic structural unit of all living things and the physical basis of all life processes; each of the body's tissues (bone, skin, muscle) is composed of many different types of cells

Central nervous system The brain and the spinal cord; controls voluntary processes such as thought and muscle movement

Chemotherapy Treatment of illness by means of chemicals (drugs)

Chromosome A small body within the nucleus of a cell that contains DNA (which in turn contains genes)

Clinical trials Medical research performed on human beings

Consent Formal, written permission to permit medical treatment; consent is a legal contract and thus cannot be executed by a person under age 18

Denial An assertion that something either does not exist or is not true; refusal to believe that which is obvious; disbelief in reality

Diagnosis Recognition of a disease from various signs and symptoms; putting a name to a medical condition

Disability An incapacity to perform one or more physical or mental tasks; a condition that prevents one from living a "normal" life with full mental, emotional, and physical function

DNA (deoxyribonucleic acid) The molecule that controls the essential life processes of all cells; it transmits cells' genetic information from one generation to the next

Emancipated minor A person under age 18 who is a parent, married, serving in the armed forces, financially independent, or otherwise living as an adult

Endocrine gland A ductless gland that produces a secretion, called a *hormone*, that is emptied into the bloodstream or lymph system and creates an effect on tissue

Excision   Removing tissue from the body

Family therapy   Psychotherapy in which the entire family participates

Fee-for-service health insurance   Also called *traditional* or *conventional insurance*; based on payment directly to health care providers by the insurance company; premiums are paid by individuals or (at least partially) by employers

Gene   A factor present in sex cells that is responsible for the transmission of hereditary characteristics

Gestational   Having to do with what happens during pregnancy, either to the mother or to the fetus

Health maintenance organization (HMO)   Managed care health insurance plan in which, for a monthly or quarterly fee (paid by the consumer or his or her employer), all health care is provided with few, if any, additional costs

Immune system   The system, composed of white blood cells, lymph, and other materials, that provides a defense against bodily invaders such as viruses, bacteria, and other organisms

Incision   Cutting into the body

Lymph   A clear body fluid, similar to plasma, that contains white blood cells and other matter; carried within a network of vessels, called the *lymph system*, that are interspersed with "pools" of collected lymph, called *nodes*

Malignant   Cancerous; also, a condition that is not necessarily cancer but that worsens until it causes death

Medicaid   A joint federal-state program that provides some health care services to people whose income is below a certain level

Medicare A federal program in which some health care services are provided to people over 65 years of age and to individuals who have been disabled more than 24 months, including children with cancer

Metastasis Spread of cancer from the original site to another place in the body

Mutation A spontaneous change in the characteristics of a gene

Neoplasm New tissue; a tumor or growth

Oncology The branch of medicine that deals with the treatment of cancer

Pediatrician Physician who specializes in the care of children

Platelets Cells that form the body's basic blood clotting mechanism; these cells react to tissue injuries

Preexisting condition A health problem that existed prior to the effective date of a health insurance policy; delineation of the conditions that apply is established by an insurance company

Prognosis The likely outcome of a disease; an educated guess

Protocol A regimen or plan of action for treating a disease or conducting medical research

Psychiatrist A medical doctor who specializes in conditions affecting the mind and emotions

Psychologist A person who holds a doctoral degree (Ph.D.) and treats conditions of the mind and emotions

Radiation A process by which energy is transmitted through space or matter; treatment with a radioactive substance

Recurrence   Reappearance of a disease; *see* Relapse

Red blood cells   Cells shaped like flat disks whose main function is to carry oxygen from the lungs to all the cells and tissues of the body; manufactured by the bone marrow

Rehabilitation   The effort to restore, maintain, or prevent further decline in body function

Relapse   Recurrence of a disease after initial treatment

Remission   Lessening of severity of a disease; abatement of symptoms

Resistance   The body's inability to respond to a certain treatment, such as a drug or radiation; diminution of or lack of effect on the disease for which the treatment is intended

Second opinion   Asking another physician to confirm or disagree with the diagnosis of a first physician; advantageous when a diagnosis is not clear-cut, when the original physician is not a specialist, or when surgery or other complex procedures are contemplated

Staging   A part of the diagnosis in which the cancer is classified according to its nature and extent of invasiveness

Stress   A condition in which psychological and/or physiological equilibrium is disrupted when a force (called a *stressor*) is exerted on something and causes change; an action that causes physical or emotional strain or deformation

Support group   A group of people, drawn together by a common problem or issue, who meet regularly to discuss the issues involved in the common concern and to solve problems that relate to it; sometimes led by a mental health professional

Sympathetic nervous system   A part of the autonomic nervous system that controls involuntary body processes such as respiration, digestion, and glandular activity

Symptom   A change in the body or its functions that indicates disease

Ultrasonography   Sound waves above the frequency detectable by the human ear that bounce off tissues to create an image of that tissue

White blood cells   Called *leukocytes*; scavengers of the bloodstream that engulf and kill invading microorganisms; a major component of the immune system

Bibliography

Adams DW, Deveau EJ: Coping with Childhood Cancer: Where Do We Go From Here? Reston, VA, Reston Publishing, 1984

Bluebond-Langner M: The Private Worlds of Dying Children. Princeton, NJ, Princeton University Press, 1978

Chesler MA, Barbarin OA: Childhood Cancer and the Family: Meeting the Challenge. New York, Brunner/Mazel, 1987

Deasy-Spinetta P, Spinetta J: The child with cancer in school: teachers' appraisal. American Journal of Pediatric Hematology/Oncology 2:89–94, 1980

Ekert H: Childhood Cancer: Understanding and Coping. New York, Gordon & Breach, 1989

Green DM: Long-Term Complications of Therapy for Cancer in Childhood and Adolescence (The Johns Hopkins Series in Contemporary Medicine and Public Health). Baltimore, MD, Johns Hopkins University Press, 1989

Green DM, D'Angio GJ: Late Effects of Treatment for Childhood Cancer. New York, Wiley-Liss, 1992

Kellerman J (ed): Psychological Aspects of Childhood Cancer. Springfield, IL, Charles C. Thomas, 1980

Koocher GP, O'Malley JE: The Damocles Syndrome: Psychosocial Consequences of Surviving Childhood Cancer. New York, McGraw-Hill, 1981

Maul-Mellott SK, Adams J: Childhood Cancer: A Nursing Overview. Boston, MA, Jones & Bartlett, 1987

McElwain TJ: Clinical management of solid tumour in childhood, in Cancer Surveys, Vol. 3 (No. 4). Oxford, UK, Oxford University Press, 1984, pp 574–752

Mullen F, Hoffman B: Charting the Journey: Almanac of Practical Resources for Cancer Survivors. Mt. Vernon, NY, Consumers Union, 1990

Noll RB, Bukowski WM, Davies WH: Peer relationships of children with cancer. Candlelighters Childhood Cancer Foundation Newsletter 16(3):1, 4, 1992

Peckham VC: Cognitive late effects of treatment, I. Candlelighters Childhood Cancer Foundation Newsletter 15(4):1, 4–5, 8, 1991

Peckham VC: Cognitive late effects of treatment, II. Candlelighters Childhood Cancer Foundation Newsletter 16(1):1, 8, 1992

Pizzo PA, Poplack DG: Principles and Practices of Pediatric Oncology. Philadelphia, PA, JB Lippincott, 1989

President's Commission for the Study of Ethical Problems in Medicine and Biomedical and Behavioral Research: Protecting Human Subjects: The Adequacy and Uniformity of Federal Rules and Their Implementation (GPO No. 040-000-00-452-1). Washington, DC, U.S. Government Printing Office, 1981

Schorr-Ribera H: Caring for siblings during diagnosis and treatment. Candlelighters Childhood Cancer Foundation Newsletter 16(2):1, 4, 1992

Van Eys J: Cancer in the Very Young. Springfield, IL, Charles C. Thomas, 1988

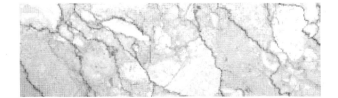

Index

Other New Harbinger Self-Help Titles